# Self-Efficacy in Nursing

*Research and*
*Measurement Perspectives*

# Editors

**Elizabeth R. Lenz, PhD, RN, FAAN** is Dean of the College of Nursing at The Ohio State University. Prior to assuming the deanship in September, 2001, she held faculty and academic administrative positions at Columbia University, The Pennsylvania State University, the University of Maryland, Georgetown University and Boston College. Lenz received her baccalaureate degree from DePauw University, Indiana, her master's degree from Boston College, and her doctorate in sociology from the University of Delaware. She is known for her work in doctoral nursing education and in nursing theory, particularly middle-range theories that inform nursing practice. Dr. Lenz's research career has focused on the family as the context for health and illness. Her most recent research concerns the outcomes and quality of nurse practitioner practice. She is on the Editorial Board of *Nursing Outlook* and between 1999 and 2001 served as an editor of *Scholarly Inquiry for Nursing Practice*.

**Lillie M. Shortridge-Baggett, EdD, RN, FAAN** is Professor and Executive Director, Center for Nursing Research, Clinical Practice and International Affairs at the Lienhard School of Nursing, Pace University. She holds joint appointments at the Division of Nursing Science, University Medical Center, Utrecht, The Netherlands and Queensland University of Technology, Brisbane, Australia. Shortridge-Baggett received her baccalaureate degree from Berea College, Kentucky, and her master's and doctoral degrees from Teachers College, Columbia University. She has been at the forefront of developments in nurse practitioner education, nurse-managed health centers, and health promotion programs. She has received numerous grants and has authored chapters, books and articles on nurse-managed care, diabetes, the use of seclusion in psychiatry, homelessness and homeless parents, collaborative health care, and collaborative research through international consortia.

## Editors, *Scholarly Inquiry for Nursing Practice*

This book was initially developed as a special issue (Volume 15, Number 3, Fall, 2001) of *Scholarly Inquiry for Nursing Practice*. The editors of the journal are listed below, with their affiliations at the time of special issue publication.

**Ruth Bernstein Hyman, PhD**
*Independent Scholar*

**Kathleen Southerton, RNC, PhD**
*SUNY Stony Brook, University Hospital and Medical Center*

**Elizabeth R. Lenz, PhD, RN, FAAN**
*Columbia University School of Nursing*

**Pierre Woog, PhD**
*Adelphi University*

# Self-Efficacy in Nursing

## Research and Measurement Perspectives

**Elizabeth R. Lenz,** PhD, FAAN
**Lillie M. Shortridge-Baggett,**
EdD, RN, FAAN, Editors

 *Springer Publishing Company*

Springer Publishing Company, Inc.
536 Broadway
New York, NY 10012-3955

*Acquisitions Editor: Ruth Chasek*
*Production Editor: Sara H. Yoo*
*Cover design by Susan Hauley*

01 02 03 04 05 / 5 4 3 2 1

**Library of Congress Cataloging-in-Publication-Data**

Self-efficacy in nursing : research and measurement perspectives / Elizabeth R. Lenz, Lillie M. Shortridge-Baggett, editors.
   p. cm.
"Originally developed as a special issue of the journal Scholarly inquiry for nursing practice."
Includes bibliographical references and index.
ISBN 0-8261-1563-2
   1. Self-efficacy.  2. Control (Psychology).  3. Nursing.  I. Lenz, Elizabeth R., 1943–  II. Shortridge-Baggett, Lillie M.

RT42.S435 2002
610.73'01'9—dc21
                                      2001059789

Printed in the United States of America by Maple-Vail Book Manufacturing Group.

# Contents

## Part III: Self-Efficacy and Other Clinical Conditions

# Contributors

**Jaap J. van der Bijl, PhD, RN**
Division of Nursing Science
University Medical Center
Utrecht, The Netherlands
Master of Science in Nursing Program
  of the Hogeschool van Utrecht
Utrecht, The Netherlands

**Linda Bunyard, RD, LD**
University of Maryland
VA Maryland Health Care System
Baltimore, MD
USA

**Norma E. Conner, MS, RN**
College of Nursing
Rutgers University
Newark, NJ
USA

**Karen M. Daley, MS, RN**
College of Nursing
Rutgers University
Newark, NJ
USA

**Karen E. Dennis, PhD, RN, FAAN**
School of Nursing
University of Central Florida
Orlando, FL
USA

**Cristina Fernandez, BS**
College of Nursing
Rutgers University
Newark, NJ
USA

**Andrew P. Goldberg, MD**
University of Maryland
VA Maryland Health Care System
Baltimore, MD
USA

**Mieke H. F. Grypdonck, PhD, RN**
University Medical Center
Utrecht, The Netherlands
University of Gent
Gent, Belgium

**Michel J. Kappen, MS, RN**
Netherlands Institute for Care and
  Welfare
Utrecht, The Netherlands

**Dorine J. E. M. Koopman-van den
  Berg, MS, RN**
Hogeschool Enschede
Enschede, The Netherlands

**Katja E. W. van de Laar, BS, RN**
University of Utrecht
Utrecht, The Netherlands

**Elise L. Lev, EdD, RN, CS**
College of Nursing
Rutgers University
Newark, NJ
USA

**Susan H. McCrone, PhD, RN**
School of Nursing
West Virginia University
Morgantown, West Virginia
USA

**Amber Moens, MS, RN**
General Hospital St. Rembert
Torhout, Belgium
University of Gent
Gent, Belgium

**Steven V. Owen, PhD**
University of Texas
Galveston, TX
USA

**Bing Bing Qi, MS**
University of Maryland
VA Maryland Health Care System
Baltimore, MD
USA

**Margaret Reith, MS, RN**
College of Nursing
Rutgers University
Newark, NJ
USA

**Naomi Tomoyasu, PhD**
Maryland Department of Health and
   Mental Hygiene
Baltimore, MD
USA

**Mary Joan Vaccaro-Olko, MS, RN,
   CS, FNP, CDE**
Endocrinology and Diabetes Associates
White Plains, NY
USA

# Prologue

The nursing profession has long viewed health promotion and disease prevention as important components of its domain. Nurse researchers continue to make major theoretical and empirical contributions to understanding the complexities of health-related behavior. Nurse scholars and clinicians have played a leadership role in developing and testing strategies to help individuals implement healthy lifestyles, often requiring difficult behavioral change. This book reports the work of a cluster of investigators in two countries—the United States and The Netherlands—who, through their research about self-efficacy, are advancing our understanding of the concept itself, ways in which it can be measured, and how it can be used to develop effective approaches to lifestyle change.

The genesis of the book was an exciting international theoretical and empirical collaboration between Lillie Shortridge-Baggett and researchers at the University of Utrecht, The Netherlands. Interested in improving the health promotion of diabetic patients, these investigators began to examine the potential of the concept of self-efficacy to inform their practice. A team approach was used to identify the theoretical underpinnings of the concept, develop and test effective measures of self-efficacy, and to test interventions to enhance the self-efficacy of adults, adolescents and children with diabetes. This work is reported in the first two sections of the book. The third section contains chapters by two teams of investigators who developed and tested efficacy-based interventions to promote the health and perceived well-being of different populations: postmenopausal women attempting to lose weight and breast cancer patients.

The book should be a valuable resource to investigators who are studying self-efficacy and those who are developing interventions to enhance health lifestyles. It also demonstrates the fruitful results of international collaboration among nurse scientists and clinicians. Importantly, it reflects a pattern of cumulative knowledge building that is so essential to the advancement to nursing as a discipline and to effective nursing practice.

ELIZABETH R. LENZ, PhD, FAAN
Editor

# Acknowledgments

This book is dedicated to the memory of Lauren Goldfarb for her initial work on the instruments and educational program development for the international collaborative project on diabetes mellitus. She did this work while a graduate student at the Lienhard School of Nursing, Pace University. Recognition is given to Koosje Guravage, a Dutch nurse, who did the first translations of the instruments from English to Dutch while she was a graduate nursing student, also at Pace University. Special thanks are given to all students, assistants, colleagues, and patients in several countries who have participated in the studies described in this book.

# Part I
# Introduction

# 1

# Self-Efficacy: Measurement and Intervention in Nursing

## Lillie M. Shortridge-Baggett

Assisting people to be as independent as possible in managing their health is an important role of health care providers. Achieving such independence often requires changing behavior, which is very challenging for individuals, their families, and professionals working with them. Many factors influence behavior change: knowledge, skills, health beliefs, attitudes, and social support. One important variable is self-efficacy, the belief of people that they can perform specific behaviors necessary to achieve their goals. The theory of self-efficacy has emerged as a way to understand and influence behavior change in all types of behaviors (Bandura, 1977, 1986, 1995, 1997), including those related to health promotion (O'Leary, 1985; Schwarzer & Fuchs, 1995; Shortridge & Rich, 1992; Strecher, McEvoy, DeVellis, Becker, & Rosenstock, 1986) and to chronic illness management (Bekkers, van Knippenberg, van den Borne, & van Berge-Henegouwen, 1996; Corbett, 1999; De Geest, Abraham, Dunbar-Jacob, & Vanhaecke, 1999; DiIorio, Faherty, & Manteuffel, 1992; Hurley & Shea, 1992; Lev, 1997; Ludlow & Gein, 1995; Pennings-van der Eerden, 1992; Taal, Rasker, Seydel, & Wiegman, 1993).

Considerable conceptual and empirical work has been carried out regarding the construct; therefore, it is quite well established at this point that one's self-efficacy influences the likelihood of behavior change.[1] Currently attention is being directed toward determining how best to measure self-efficacy for different behaviors and in different clinical populations and to develop programs with effective intervention strategies to improve self-efficacy. These topics are the focus of this book.

Two characteristics of the book are of particular note. First, an international focus is apparent in that five of the chapters report the results of an international collaboration between the author of this chapter and researchers in The Netherlands. This collaborative activity was focused on the measurement of self-efficacy in diabetic populations of various ages and on intervention strategies to increase self-efficacy and thus to enhance self-management behaviors in these populations. Second, with the exception of the introductory overview of the theoretical underpinnings for and measurement of the construct, the articles reflect direct practice relevance. Four chapters relate to self-efficacy in the management of diabetes in various age groups, one addresses self-efficacy in a program to encourage weight loss in postmenopausal women, and one reports the results of an intervention to increase self-efficacy of breast cancer patients.

The book begins with a review of the theoretical basis for the role of self-efficacy in changing behavior by van der Bijl and Shortidge-Baggett, who also discuss the measurement of self-efficacy in general and more specifically in diabetic populations. As discussed in this overview, the expectation that a certain behavior will have a desired outcome (outcome expectations) and that one can perform the task (efficacy expectations) should lead to the person's attempting the behavior and persisting when difficulties are encountered. People's confidence in or perception of their ability to carry out tasks directly relates to their success.

The four sources of self-efficacy information are performance accomplishments, vicarious experience, verbal persuasion, and physiological and emotional states (Bandura, 1995). Since all four sources of self-efficacy can be used to enhance self-efficacy for specific behaviors, attention needs to be given to each in developing and testing nursing interventions.

## SELF-EFFICACY INSTRUMENT DEVELOPMENT

The development of valid and reliable instruments to measure self-efficacy has been, and remains, an ongoing challenge. Of particular import in nursing is the measurement of self-efficacy in executing the behaviors needed for self-management by patients with chronic illnesses. Appropriate instruments need to be developed for specific conditions, for a variety of developmental levels, and in patients' native languages before an educational intervention can be implemented and studied (McDermott & Palchanes, 1992; Oettingen, 1995).

The development and testing of instruments to measure self-efficacy in management of diabetes mellitus are described in several of the chapters in this book. The results of studies from the international collaborative program by Kappen and colleagues and Moens and associates are included as examples of instrument development. A brief overview of the instrument development and testing process of the collaborative project is provided as background for the chapters in this book.

Initially, four Likert-type scales were developed in English, each targeted toward a different type 1 diabetic population: children, adolescents, adult diabetics, and their significant others. After content validation was completed, the scales were administered to assess reliability. The first scales to be developed in Dutch were for type 2 adult diabetics and their significant others; and later, measurement approaches and scales appropriate for children and adolescents were added. The items were generated by review of English and Dutch literature, a qualitative study of adolescent perceptions, and interviews with nurses and diabetes educators. Language problems were encountered; for example, there is no specific word for "confidence" in Dutch, so several items needed to be rewritten. Also, several of the items that seemed to be related more to "knowing" something than to behavior were reworded, replaced, or omitted (see Maibach & Murphy, 1995). Additionally, some behavioral items were updated to keep current with changes in practice. Psychometric assessment of these instruments included a more rigorous process for assessing content validity than was used in the earlier (English language) phase of instrument development (Lynn, 1986). The results of the initial development and testing of the instruments are reported in this book.

It is anticipated that all scales should continue to be tested when used with other populations to further validate each of them. Several investigators from different countries have requested permission to use the scales developed and tested in this collaborative project in their research. Permission has been granted for each request with the requirement that the results of further psychometric testing be shared with the research team and that their publications indicate that permission was granted; reprints of the articles are to be shared with the research team.

## INTERVENTION STRATEGIES
## FOR SELF-EFFICACY

Effective intervention programs are essential for persons to learn the necessary knowledge and skills required for self-management. An important part of providing an effective program for management of chronic illnesses is the development and testing of theory-based intervention strategies to enhance self-efficacy. According to Peyrot (1999), "Empirical studies of how education produces behavior change are few, but much preliminary work has been done to identify potential behavioral determinants that can be targeted by interventions. Theoretical models of behavior change have been advanced (e.g., stages of change) but they have yet to be rigorously tested" (p. 62).

Four of the chapters in this book address aspects of theory-based nursing interventions. As part of the international collaboration described above, literature about enhancing self-efficacy in patients with chronic illnesses was reviewed and strategies specific to diabetes education are summarized by van de Laar and van der Bijl. Additionally, educational programs in the Netherlands were reviewed to determine which strategies are currently being used to enhance self-efficacy. The results of this review are reported by Koopman-van den Berg and van der Bijl. Two chapters address the effectiveness of specific interventions based on self-efficacy theory. Dennis and associates discuss the use of interventions based on Bandura's theory of self-efficacy and report the success of theory-based strategies at effecting positive change in weight loss, eating behaviors, and physical conditioning. In their study of patients with breast cancer, Lev, Daley, Conner, Reith, and Fernandez examined the impact of theory-based intervention strategies based on quality of life, perceived self-care, self-efficacy and symptoms.

# SUMMARY

Assisting people with chronic illnesses to change their behavior is important in effecting self-management and in achieving the highest possible level of health. There is increasing evidence that a vital ingredient in health-related behavior change is the perceived self-efficacy of the individual to behave differently; however, disease- and age-specific measures and interventions have received insufficient attention to date. This book reports the results of the first stages of an international collaboration that is addressing the development and testing of instruments and interventions to measure and ultimately to enhance self-efficacy in management of diabetes mellitus. These instruments are now being used and tested further by other investigators, as well as in ongoing studies by the authors. Additionally, the book addresses the importance of theory-based interventions and their use in enhancing self-efficacy as a means of encouraging positive behavior change. The results of two intervention studies designed to improve patients' self-management of obesity and cancer support the use of strategies to enhance self-efficacy in changing behavior. They also underscore the need to continue to identify, develop and test targeted nursing interventions.

# NOTE

[1]An excellent overview of self-efficacy is included on a special web page on Bandura established by Pajares (2000) at Emory University: www.emory.edu/ EDUCATION/mfp/effpage.html. Included are a general introduction to the concept, overviews of self-efficacy theory, measures and current research directions, and the following aspects and areas of application: career/occupational factors; computers/media interactivity/technology; health behaviors; organizational/administrative/managerial factors; personality factors; schooling; social/cultural factors; and sports.

# REFERENCES

Bandura, A. (1977). Self-efficacy: Toward a unifying theory of behavior change. *Psychological Review, 84*(2), 191-192.

Bandura, A. (1986). *Social foundations of thought and action: A social cognitive theory.* Englewood Cliffs, NJ: Prentice Hall.

Bandura, A. (1995). Exercise of personal and collective efficacy in changing societies. In A. Bandura (Ed.), *Self-efficacy in changing societies* (pp. 1-45). New York: Press Syndicate of the University of Cambridge.

Bandura, A. (1997). *Self-efficacy: The exercise of control.* New York: Freeman.

Bekkers, J. T. M., van Knippenberg, F. C. E., van den Borne, H. W., & van Berge-Henegouwen, G. P. (1996). Prospective evaluation of psychosocial adaptation to stoma surgery: The role of self-efficacy. *Psychosomatic Medicine, 58,* 183-191.

Bijl, J. J. van der, Poelgeest-Eeltink, A. van, & Shortridge-Baggett, L. M. (1998). De psychometriche eigenschappen van de self-efficacy schaal voor niet-insuline-afhankelijke diabeten [Psychometric properties of the self-efficacy scale for non-insulin dependent diabetic]. *Verpleegkunde, 13*(1), 15-24.

Bijl, J. J. van der, Poelgeest-Eeltink, A. van, & Shortridge-Baggett, L. M. (1999). Psychometric properties of the diabetes management self-efficacy scale for patients with type 2 diabetes mellitus. *Journal of Advanced Nursing, 30*(2), 352-359.

Brown, S. A. (1999). Interventions to promote diabetes self-management: State of the science. *The Diabetes Educator, 25*(Suppl. 6), 52-61.

Corbett, C. F. (1999). Research-based practice implications for patients with diabetes. *Home Healthcare Nurse, 17,* 587-596.

De Geest, S., Abraham, I., Dunbar-Jacob, J., & Vanhaecke, J. (1999). Behavioral strategies for long-term survival of transplant recipients. In J. M. Metry & U. A. Meyer (Eds.), *Drug regimen compliance: Issues in clinical trials and patient management* (pp. 163-179). New York: Wiley.

DiIorio, C., Faherty, B., & Manteuffel, B. (1992). Self-efficacy and social support in self-management of epilepsy. *Western Journal of Nursing Research, 14*(3), 292-307.

Fain, J. A., Nettles, A., Funnell, M. M., & Charron, D. (1999). Diabetes patient education research: An integrative literature review. *The Diabetes Educator, 25* (Suppl. 6), 7-15.

Glasgow, R. E. (1999). Outcomes of and for diabetes education research. *The Diabetes Educator, 25*(Suppl. 6), 74-88.

Hurley, A. C., & Shea, C. A. (1992). Self-efficacy: Strategy for enhancing diabetes self-care. *The Diabetes Educator, 18*(2), 146-150.

Lev, E. L. (1997). Bandura's theory of self-efficacy: Applications to oncology. *Scholarly Inquiry for Nursing Practice: An International Journal, 11,* 21-37.

Ludlow, A., & Gein, L. (1995). Relationship among self-care, self-efficacy and HbA1c levels in individuals with noninsulin dependent diabetes mellitus (NIDDM). *Canadian Journal of Diabetes Care, 19*(1), 10-15.

Lynn, M. (1986). Determination and quantification of content validity. *Nursing Research, 35*(6), 382-385.

Maibach, E., & Murphy, D. A. (1995). Self-efficacy in health promotion research and practice: Conceptualization and measurement. *Health Education Research, 10* (1), 37-50.

McDermott, A. N., & Palchanes, K. (1992). A process for translating and testing a quantitative measure for cross-cultural nursing research. *Journal of the New York State Nurses Association, 23,* 12-15.

Oettingen, G. (1995). Cross-cultural perspectives on self-efficacy. In A. Bandura (Ed.), *Self-efficacy in changing societies* (pp.149-176). New York: Cambridge University Press.

O'Leary, A. (1985). Self-efficacy and health. *Behavior Research and Therapy, 23,* 437-451.

Pajares, F. (2000, February 2). *Current directions in self-efficacy research* [Online]. Available: www.emory.edu/EDUCATION/mfp/effchapter.html

Pennings-van der Eerden, L. (1992). *Self-care behavior in the treatment of diabetes mellitus* (Doctoral dissertation, University of Utrecht). Amsterdam: Thesis Publishers.

Peyrot, M. (1999). Behavior change in diabetes education. *The Diabetes Educator, 25* (Suppl. 6), 62-73.

Schwarzer, R., & Fuchs, R. (1995). Self-efficacy and health behaviours. In M. Conner & P. Norman (Eds.), *Predicting health behavior: Research and practice with social cognition models.* Buckingham: Open University Press.

Shortridge, L. M. (1994). Nursing research from a Dutch perspective. In J. J. Fitzpatrick, H. S. Sternson, & E. Tomquist (Eds.), *Nursing research and its utilization: International state of the science* (pp. 217-221). New York: Springer Publishing.

Shortridge, L. M., & Rich, E. (1992). *Personal health management program.* Pleasantville, NY: Pace University.

Shortridge-Baggett, L. M., & van der Bijl, J. (1996). International collaborative research on management self-efficacy in diabetes mellitus. *The Journal of the New York State Nurses Association, 27,* 9-14.

Shortridge-Baggett, L. M. (1999, October). *Establishing an international collaborative program of nursing research.* Paper presented at the Distinguished Nurse Researcher Award Luncheon of the Foundation of the New York State Nurses Association, Lake Placid, NY.

Strecher, V. J., McEvoy, De Vellis, Becker, M., & Rosenstock, L. M. (1986). The role of self-efficacy in achieving health behavior change. *Health Education Quarterly, 13*(1), 73-91.

Taal, E., Rasker, J., Seydel, E., & Wiegman, O. (1993). Health status, adherence with health recommendations, self-efficacy and social support in patients with rheumatoid arthritis. *Patient Education and Counseling, 20*(2/3), 63-76.

# 2

# The Theory and Measurement of the Self-Efficacy Construct

## Jaap J. van der Bijl
## Lillie M. Shortridge-Baggett

The purpose of this chapter is to provide:

1. Overviews of the literature on the theoretical background of self-efficacy, its determinants and consequences and the way self-efficacy is supposed to be measured in general, and
2. An illustration of the measurement issues of self-efficacy when applied to the behavioral domain of diabetes management.

The construct of self-efficacy was first introduced by Albert Bandura, a psychologist, who used Social Learning Theory (later labeled as Social Cognitive Theory) as a conceptual basis for analysis of this construct (Bandura, 1977). Social Cognitive Theory represents a triadic reciprocal causation model in which the behavior of a person, the characteristics of that person, and the environment within which the behavior is performed are constantly interacting (Bandura, 1977, 1986). Thus, behavior is not simply the result of the environment and the person, just as the environment is not simply the result of the person and behavior. A change in one component has implications for the others. For example, if an individual has lost a job during a recessionary period, lack of money will influence his or her behavior and well-being (Bandura, 1995).

Dealing with one's environment involves, according to Bandura (1986), a complex set of behaviors. Cognitive, social, and behavioral subskills must be organized into integrated courses of action to exercise some control over events that affect people's lives. It is Bandura's conviction, supported by an increasing number of research findings from diverse fields, that the effective use and execution of these subskills is strongly related to people's beliefs of personal efficacy in executing these skills. The influential role of judgments of personal efficacy was, after its introduction in 1977, further explored by Bandura under the name, self-efficacy (Bandura, 1986, 1997a).

# SELF-EFFICACY

## Definition of Self-Efficacy

Perceived self-efficacy (henceforth, self-efficacy) is defined as "people's judgments of their capabilities to organize and execute courses of action required to attain designated types of performances. It is concerned not with the skills one has but with judgments of what one can do with whatever skills one possesses" (Bandura, 1986, p. 391). This description shows that people's self-efficacy is not of a general nature, but related to specific situations. Individuals can judge themselves to be very competent in a specific field and less competent in another field. For instance, a person can be convinced that he or she is able to run 10 kilometers but be quite certain he or she is not able to run a marathon. This means that self-efficacy is related to specific situations and tasks, which is not the case for related concepts like self-esteem, self-confidence and locus of control (Maibach & Murphy, 1995). Unlike self-efficacy, these are personal characteristics of individuals which have a certain stable influence on people's behavior. In other words, for each individual it can be established whether he or she has much or little self-confidence, but not whether this individual generally has a high or low measure of self-efficacy. No global sense of self-efficacy exists. Thus, self-efficacy is not a personality trait, but a temporary and easy to influence characteristic that is strictly situation- and task-related.

## Self-Efficacy Theory

The basic premise underlying self-efficacy theory according to Bandura (1977, 1986) is that the expectations of personal mastery (efficacy expectations or self-efficacy) and success (outcome expectations) determine whether an individual will engage in a particular behavior. Together with the characteristics of a person, the behavior of the person and the outcomes of the behavior, these two kinds of expectations, efficacy expectations and outcome expectations, form Bandura's model of self-efficacy theory (see Figure 2.1). An outcome expectation is a person's belief about the outcomes that result from a given behavior. These outcomes can take the form of physical, social or self-evaluative effects. An efficacy expectation, or self-efficacy, concerns the confidence in one's capability to produce the behavior. People are motivated to perform behaviors they believe will produce desired outcomes. Outcome expectations are highly dependent, however, on efficacy expectations (self-efficacy) and therefore, self-efficacy predicts performance much better than expected outcomes (Bandura, 1986).

## Sources of Self-Efficacy

Self-efficacy beliefs are influenced by four important sources of information: performance accomplishments, vicarious experience, verbal persuasion, and physiological information (Bandura, 1977, 1986, 1995, 1997a).

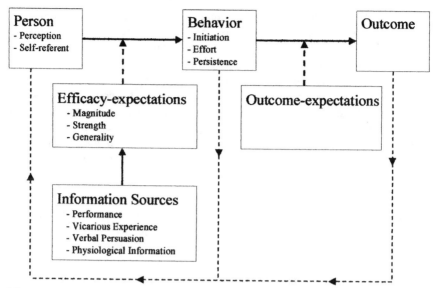

**Figure 2.1.** Self-efficacy model (Shortridge-Baggett & van der Bijl, 1996).

***Performance Accomplishments: Practicing and Earlier Experiences.*** Practicing is the most important source of self-efficacy because it is based on a person's own experience. Experiences of success (the feeling of mastery) enhance self-efficacy, while regular failure decreases self-efficacy, especially when the failure takes place early in the learning process. Once a person has developed a strong self-efficacy, one failure does not have much influence. The effects of failure depend on the moment in the learning process and the total pattern of experiences. Once a person has high self-efficacy, she or he tends to generalize from one experience to another, with the obvious danger that the skills from the former experience are not always relevant to the latter. Experience with behavior and the attributions of success and failure are an important source for the development of expectations of efficacy. Persons who are certain of their capacities tend to attribute failure to situational factors like not enough effort or bad strategy. Persons with low self-efficacy will sooner attribute failure to their own incapacity.

***Vicarious Experience: Observation of Others.*** Seeing others perform successfully also is an important source of self-efficacy. Other persons can serve as examples (role models) and supply information about the degree of difficulty of a specific kind of behavior. The people serving as role models, however, should show similarity to the observer in those characteristics which are relevant to the issue. In some situations persons are extra sensitive to observed information. In case of uncertainty about one's own capacities or inexperience with a specific kind of behavior, people use observed indicators by which they can measure their own capacities and on which they can base their estimation of success. Observing others is a weaker source of self-efficacy than direct experience, but can contribute to a person's judgment of his or her own self-efficacy.

***Verbal Persuasion.*** Verbal persuasion is the most often used source of self-efficacy, because it is easy to use. By giving instructions, suggestions and advice, health care professionals try to convince persons that they can succeed in a difficult task. Of critical importance are the credibility, expertise, trustworthiness, and prestige of the person doing the persuasion. Verbal attempts to convince people that they have the ability to perform a behavior are weaker than the previous two sources because they do not concern one's own experiences or examples of them. Persuasion can be a good supplementation to other sources, however. If people are convinced of their abilities, they will be more inclined to persevere and will not give up easily. This is only the case, however, with persons who already think they are able to carry out a task and is useless if it is not realistic.

***Physiological Information: Self-Evaluation of Physiological and Emotional States.*** Information on the human body can also influence a person's estimation of the capability to show a specific behavior. In judging their own capacities persons use information about their physiological and emotional situations. They experience tension, anxiety, and depression as signs of personal deficiency. In activities that require strength and perseverance, they interpret fatigue, pain, hypoglycaemia as indicators of low physical efficacy. Persons expect to be more successful when they are not stressed than when they are. Stress can have a negative influence on self-efficacy. What persons believe about their illness and how they interpret their symptoms influences their self-efficacy to deal with the illness.

The self-efficacy from the different sources needs to be processed cognitively. Many factors influence the cognitive estimation of experiences, for instance, personal, situational, social and time factors. In forming a judgment of efficacy persons have to weigh and integrate information from the different sources (Bandura, 1986).

A certain hierarchy exists in the four information sources of self-efficacy. The first source, the repeated execution of the task, is the most powerful source because it is based on direct information: people immediately experience success or failure. The other three sources are all based on indirect information. Modeling, seeing other people demonstrate the desired behavior, can offer very important self-efficacy information but is not based on one's own experiences. Persuasion is a weaker source, especially when used by itself. This source usually is used to support the other sources. The last source, the physiological information, is the least concrete. People rely on their physical and emotional states to judge their capabilities (Bandura, 1997a; Schunk & Carbonari, 1984).

***Other Sources of Self-Efficacy.*** Besides the four previously described sources of self-efficacy, other factors can have their effect on self-efficacy. Strecher, DeVellis, Becker, and Rosenstock (1986) state that personality traits, states and processes can influence self-efficacy expectations. They refer to several concepts closely linked to self-efficacy: locus of control, self-esteem, self-confidence and hardiness. Studies have confirmed the relationship between self-efficacy and other personal factors. Coppel (1980), for example, found a positive relationship between self-esteem and self-efficacy, and Schneewind (1995) reported that people with an internal locus of control had high self-efficacy.

Furthermore, environmental factors like expectations and support of others can have an effect on self-efficacy (Bandura, 1986). The presence of social support in the form of instrumental support or persuasive communication is helpful in overcoming obstacles in the pursuit of behavioral goals. The relationship between support received from others and self-efficacy has been demonstrated (e.g., DiIorio, Faherty, & Manteuffel, 1994; Talbot, Nouwen, Gringas, Gosselin, & Audet, 1997).

In their theoretical analysis of the determinants of self-efficacy, Gist and Mitchel (1992) especially focus on the causal processes and information cues involved in the formation of self-efficacy as elaborated in attribution theory (Weiner, 1979, 1985). Gist and Mitchel suggest that the experiences of mastery, modeling, persuasion, and physiological information are more complex than their labels imply. Each of these experiences contributes a variety of external and internal information cues that can influence self-efficacy.

Internal information cues refer to the individual's ability (knowledge and skills) and the effectiveness of various performance strategies that utilize these skills. Self-efficacy will be determined, in part, by the person's assessment of whether his or her abilities are adequate, inferior or superior for performance at various task levels. Individuals also make judgments about anticipated performance based on how positively aroused (i.e., excited, enthusiastic) or negatively aroused (i.e., fearful, anxious) they feel when confronted with a particular task. This arousal may be influenced by the individual's general health condition, personality (e.g., type A or B personality), and mood. Kavanagh and Bower (1985), for example, demonstrated that a mood manipulation resulted in higher self-efficacy scores for a positive mood and lower self-efficacy scores for a negative mood.

External information cues refer to the task itself. First, the task attributes are important. Estimates of self-efficacy may include considerations of the degree of interdependence and the amount of resources (i.e., material resources, time, and social support) required to complete the task successfully. Another external information cue related to any task is its complexity. In the formation of self-efficacy, the important components of complexity include the number of component parts involved in completing the task, uncertainty, and the sequential or coordinative steps required to perform the task successfully. The task's environment also may influence performance estimates. A task environment in which there are many distractions (e.g., noise and interruptions) may lower performance estimates when compared with a task environment that is less distracting. Also, the amount of risk or danger in the setting may influence self-efficacy. Other external factors that may relate to self-efficacy are physical conditions like the weather or the geographic setting (e.g., the safe environment of the home versus the more risky environment of school or work).

In addition to these internal personal factors and external environmental factors which may influence self-efficacy, Gist and Mitchel (1992) stress the importance of considering the variability (over time and occasions) and the controllability of the self-efficacy determinant. When making self-efficacy assessments, individuals consider the level of variability (low or high) of the determinants and also whether they exercise control over the determinants. Some factors are primarily under personal control (such as effort) and some are primarily under the control of others (like the willingness to give support). In many cases, individuals have little or no control or influence over external factors. Thus, perceived control is likely to be higher over internal than external factors. Regarding variability, some factors can change immediately (such as knowledge), whereas others may be changeable, but only after a long period of time (such as ability or general physical condition). Thus, perceived control may be higher over determinants that are immediately variable than over those that are relatively more stable.

The more people believe that the causes of performance are uncontrollable and possess a low level of variability, the lower and more resistant to change will be their self-efficacy. Therefore, a good understanding of both the task and the individual is needed if self-efficacy is to be enhanced.

## THE CONSEQUENCES OF SELF-EFFICACY

Self-efficacy theory suggests that self-efficacy, people's beliefs in their abilities to perform specific behaviors, is an important predictor of how they are functioning in terms of choice behavior, effort expenditure and persistence, thought patterns and emotional reactions. In other words self-efficacy influences how people think, feel, motivate themselves, and act. Self-efficacy thus contributes to the quality of psychosocial functioning in diverse ways (Bandura, 1986).

### Choice Behavior or Selection Processes

Every day people make decisions about what activities to pursue or to avoid. Decisions involving choice of activities are influenced by judgments of self-efficacy. People tend to avoid tasks and situations they believe exceed their capabilities, while pursuing those they feel competent to perform (Bandura, 1977, 1986). For example, persons with diabetes with a low sense of self-efficacy in diabetes management behavior shy away from difficult tasks, such as monitoring blood glucose levels or sticking to their diabetes diet, which they view as personal threats (Hockmeyer, 1990). In contrast, people with diabetes with a high sense of self-efficacy approach these difficult tasks as challenges to be mastered rather than threats to be avoided.

### Effort Expenditure and Persistence of Motivational Processes

People motivate themselves by forming beliefs about what they can do, anticipating likely outcomes, setting goals, and planning courses of action. Their motivation will be stronger if they believe they can attain their goals and adjust them based on their progress. Individuals who have a high level of self-efficacy are more persistent in the face of difficulties than those with a lower level of self-efficacy. Also, in the case of failures or setbacks, people with low self-efficacy tend to give up or reduce their effort, whereas those with high self-efficacy generally intensify their efforts until they succeed (Bandura & Cervone, 1983).

## Thought Patterns or Cognitive Processes

Self-efficacy also affects thought patterns that can enhance or undermine performance. These cognitive processes take three forms (Bandura, 1995; Maibach & Murphy, 1995):

1. Goals and aspirations: the stronger the self-efficacy, the higher the goal challenges people set for themselves and the firmer their commitment to them.
2. Visualization of positive and negative performance scenarios: those who have a high sense of self-efficacy visualize success scenarios that provide positive guides and supports for performance. Those with low self-efficacy visualize failure scenarios and dwell on the many things that can go wrong.
3. Quality of analytical thinking: high self-efficacy encourages analytical thought processes in reaction to setbacks and difficulties.

## Emotional Effects or Affective Processes

People's beliefs in their coping capabilities affect how much stress and depression they experience in threatening or difficult situations, as well as their level of motivation. Self-efficacy regulates emotional states in several ways (Bandura, 1995):

1. People who believe they can manage threats are less distressed by them; those who lack self-efficacy are more likely to magnify risks;
2. People with high self-efficacy lower their stress and anxiety by acting in ways that make the environment less threatening;
3. People with high coping capacities have better control over disturbing thoughts; and
4. Low self-efficacy can lead directly to depression.

In summary, people's self-efficacy influences the choices they make, their aspirations, the amount of exertion they put in to reach certain goals, how long they can persevere in case of setbacks or failures, their thinking patterns, the experienced amount of stress and their susceptibility to depression.

It is hypothesized, therefore, that self-efficacy plays an important role in predicting behavior and its outcomes (Bandura, 1986). This hypothesis has received support from a growing body of research findings from diverse fields.

Self-efficacy has been found to be related to a wide range of clinical problems (Pajares, 1997).

## MEASUREMENT OF SELF-EFFICACY
## IN GENERAL

Bandura (1977) indicates that the concept of self-efficacy has three dimensions, that is, magnitude (or level), strength and generality. Magnitude refers to how difficult a person finds it to adopt a specific behavior. Strength reflects how certain a person is of being able to perform a specific task. Generality refers to the degree to which self-efficacy beliefs are positively related, either within a behavioral domain, across behavioral domains or across time. Self-efficacy is then measured by obtaining ratings of strength, magnitude and generality.

Although Bandura (1997a) is very specific about the level of specificity at which perceived self-efficacy should be measured, others (e.g., Schwarzer, 1993) have developed instruments to assess self-efficacy at a more general personality level than Bandura advocates. They argue that broader and more general dispositional measures are usually better suited for predicting more general patterns of behavior or outcomes that arise across multiple contexts (Smith, Wallston, & Smith, 1995). Bandura (1997a), however, has cautioned researchers that, to increase accuracy of prediction, "self-efficacy beliefs should be measured in terms of particularized judgments of capability that may vary across realms of activity, different levels of task demands within a given activity domain, and under different situational circumstances" (p. 6). In his view efficacy beliefs should be assessed at the optimal level of specificity that corresponds to the criterion task being assessed and the domain of functioning being analyzed. Maibach and Murphy (1995) argue that some researchers have incorrectly interpreted generality of self-efficacy to mean generalized self-efficacy, that is, a sense of efficacy that operates across all situations and domains of functioning. Treating generality of self-efficacy in this fashion distorts the self-efficacy construct as described by Bandura. The problem with assessments of generalized self-efficacy is that people must make judgments about their capabilities without a clear activity or task in mind. Therefore, general self-efficacy instruments have little explanatory and predictive value in contrast to domain-related measures (Pajares, 1997).

The construction of sound self-efficacy scales relies on a good conceptual analysis of the relevant domain of functioning (Bandura, 1997b). Knowledge of the activity domain allows one to specify which aspects of self-efficacy should be measured. A comprehensive assessment of self-efficacy would be linked to the behavioral factors over which people can exercise some control. Behavior is better predicted by people's beliefs in their capabilities to do whatever is needed to succeed than by their beliefs in only one aspect of self-efficacy relevant to the domain. Consider the self-management of weight as an example. Weight is determined by what people eat, by their level of exercise, and genetic factors. In this example, perceived self-efficacy will account for more of the variation in weight if the assessment includes perceived capability to regulate food purchases, eating habits and exercise than if it is confined solely to eating habits. The self-efficacy items should accurately reflect the construct under investigation. Self-efficacy is concerned with perceived capability. The items should be phrased in terms of *can do* rather than *will do*. *Can* is a judgment of capability; *will* is a statement of intention.

The traditional measurement of self-efficacy (Bandura, 1997b; Maibach & Murphy, 1995) started from the idea that an individual responds dichotomously (yes or no) to whether he or she is capable of performing a specific task at various levels of difficulty. The sum of positive responses is the magnitude of self-efficacy. For each affirmative response, confidence is then rated on a 100-point scale, ranging in 10-unit intervals from 10 ("Little certainty") through intermediate degrees of assurance, 50 ("Moderately certain can do") to complete assurance, 100 ("Highly certain"). The sum of confidence ratings is the strength of self-efficacy. A second and more common and convenient approach to self-efficacy assessment incorporates the two judgments (can/cannot do and confidence rating) into a single item using a 0 to 100-point scale anchored at one end with "Cannot do at all" (0) and at the other end with "Certain can do" (100). This produces efficacy ratings equivalent to the two-question format. The self-efficacy scores are summed and divided by the total number of items to indicate the strength of perceived self-efficacy for different levels of performance (magnitude) regarding the activity domain under investigation. An illustration of this latter approach is presented in Figure 2.2.

Some researchers retain the same scale structure and descriptors but use single unit intervals ranging from 0 to 10. On some occasions, Likert-type scales have been used which simply ask how well the person thinks he or she can do the task (Bandura, 1997b; Maibach & Murphy, 1995). For an example of the Likert-type self-efficacy scale, see the paragraph about measurement of diabetes management self-efficacy.

---

*"The attached form lists different activities. In the column **Confidence**, rate how confident you are that you can do them **as of now**. Rate your degree of confidence by recording a number from 0 to 100 using the scale given below."*

| 0 | 10 | 20 | 30 | 40 | 50 | 60 | 70 | 80 | 90 | 100 |
|---|----|----|----|----|----|----|----|----|----|-----|
| Cannot do at all | | | | Moderately certain can do | | | | | | Certain can do |

---

**Figure 2.2.** Example of a response format, including instructions, of a self-efficacy scale (Bandura, 1997b).

Bandura (1997a) specified a third relevant measurement dimension of self-efficacy, generality. Generality of self-efficacy, as stated before, refers to the degree to which self-efficacy beliefs are positively related, either within the domain, across behavioral domains or across time. Generality is evaluated by measuring self-efficacy beliefs over the dimensions of concern. For example, to assess the within-domain generality of self-efficacy to manage diabetes diet, diet self-efficacy is measured with reference to adjusting diet when ill and with reference to adjusting diet in case of stress. Between-domain generality is concerned with the relationship of self-efficacy beliefs across related domains of behavior, for example, perceived self-efficacy to control blood sugar level and perceived self-efficacy to inject insulin. An example of self-efficacy assessment of generality across time is given by Maibach and Murphy (1995). They refer to a study conducted by Maibach and colleagues in which the researchers assessed the generality of exercise self-efficacy across time by determining participants' current confidence to maintain a regular exercise regimen (at least three times per week) over the course of progressively longer periods of time (i.e., 1 week, 1 month, 1 year).

According to Maibach and Murphy (1995) the generality dimension of self-efficacy has not received adequate attention in health promotion research. Most health promotion studies measure only the strength dimension of self-efficacy. They state that it is not always necessary to measure all three dimensions of self-efficacy and that the purpose of the research will determine which dimensions are required. In their observation, health promotion researchers often try to measure too much with too little.

## MEASUREMENT OF DIABETES MANAGEMENT SELF-EFFICACY

Bandura (1997a) claims that self-efficacy should be assessed at the optimal level of specificity that corresponds to the specific task being assessed and the domain of functioning being analyzed. In this paragraph experiences with measurement issues of self-efficacy regarding a specific behavioral domain, diabetes management, will be presented and discussed.

When we began, we decided to develop a diabetes management self-efficacy scale measuring the strength dimension of self-efficacy among people with type 2 diabetes. This decision was based on recognition that including the other two dimensions would lead to an unacceptably long instrument, and further, Bandura (1997a) has stated that the strength dimension is most influential. The strength dimension appeared to be a reliable measure to test the impact of self-efficacy on diabetes management. The measure of self-efficacy strength we used was a 5-point semantically anchored Likert-scale (1 = yes, definitely; 2 = probably yes; 3 = maybe yes, maybe no; 4 = probably no; 5 = no, definitely not) measuring the degree of confidence of people with type 2 diabetes in diabetes management behaviors, such as checking blood sugar (van der Bijl, van Poelgeest, & Shortridge-Baggett, 1999).

Experiences in the development and testing of the self-efficacy scale for children with diabetes, however, showed us the need to incorporate the magnitude dimension (the level of difficulty of the task). The children had high self-efficacy scores but these scores were not correlated with metabolic control (HbA1c) or the diabetes nurses' assessment of the children's adherence to recommended diabetes self-care activities (Kappen, 1998). We concluded that the scale was subject to ceiling effects and that therefore the predictive validity of the scale was question-able. Interviews with parents and children revealed that the items measuring the strength of self-efficacy for various diabetes behaviors lacked sufficient challenge. For children who have had diabetes for several years, it is no big deal to inject insulin three times a day. These activities have become routine. No wonder ceiling effects were found in the perceived self-efficacy of both the children and parents.

From this we learned that measuring the strength dimension of self-efficacy serves the purpose in the case of newly diagnosed people with diabetes mellitus. When people have a history of diabetes, however, it is important to measure the magnitude dimension of self-efficacy using items that tap the complexity of the behavior or the level of challenge (Maibach & Murphy, 1995). To determine the complexity of behaviors and which behaviors are challenging, researchers should ask members of the population of interest; they are the experts. The relevant behaviors will not be revealed through content validation by an expert panel of diabetes nurses (Kappen, 1998). Maibach and Murphy therefore recommend focus group interviews and other elicitation procedures with the target population. In developing the diabetes management self-efficacy scale for adolescents, we followed this advice and, by means of focus group interviews, collected a list of relevant diabetes management behaviors for this group.

## Target Population Issues

Although different groups of people with diabetes face more or less the same daily requirements of self-care activities to reduce the risk of complications, the complexity, circumstances and challenges of diabetes management behaviors differ as a result of differences in the type of diabetes mellitus, experience with diabetes, culture group and age. These differences must be considered in identify-ing the relevant diabetes management behaviors to be reflected in a self-efficacy scale.

*Type of Diabetes Mellitus.* There are two main types of diabetes: type 1 and type 2 (Peltenburg, 1995). Type 1 and type 2 diabetes are distinct syndromes. To obtain an acceptable level of blood glucose, the person with type 1 diabetes has to inject insulin daily. Without insulin the patient will slip into a diabetic coma and eventually die. Persons with type 2 diabetes are not dependent on insulin injections. They can control the disease with diet, exercise and oral medication. Although both types of diabetes mellitus are chronic, type 1 has short-term complications that require immediate treatment, whereas type 2 has long-term complications. Type 1 is clearly manifest as a disease because of the need for regular insulin injections; type 2 can exist without being detected. Given the complex self-regulative activities for persons with type 1, it is not surprising that the complexity and challenge of diabetes management behaviors for people with type 1 differ from those for people with type 2.

A third type of diabetes mellitus is gestational diabetes mellitus, which occurs during pregnancy. Most of the time this type of diabetes disappears after delivery. Awareness that gestational diabetes is not a chronic condition means that pregnant women appraise the diabetes regimen quite differently from people with lifelong diabetes. Thus, diabetes task demands and circumstances would lead to different content for the self-efficacy scale.

*Culture.* Language differences may be important. For example, most self-efficacy instruments in the English language use the phrase: "How confident are you at . . ." (Maibach & Murphy, 1995). In Dutch, the equivalent phrases are "I think I'm able to . . . " and "Do you succeed in . . ." (Schaalma, 1993), or "To what extent do you estimate it realizable to . . ." (De Geest, 1996), or "I'm sure/certain I can . . ." (Taal, 1995), and "I'm convinced I can . . . ." (Moens, 1998). The reason for the differences in terminology is that there is no good Dutch equivalent of the concept of "confidence." In this case, however, analysis of the different terminology showed no significant distinctions (see the section about instrument format and terminology issues).

*Age.* People differ in the degree of their self-efficacy, depending on their stage of development. Physical abilities, psychological competencies, and social skills enable most people to increase the number of domains in which they can exert self-efficacy as they mature and their control over their lives increases (Flammer, 1995).

In developing diabetes management self-efficacy scales for different age-groups, these differences must be taken into account. In the development of the self-efficacy scale for children with diabetes, aged 8-12, one question was: "At what age are children able to make a valid assessment of their capacities?" (Kappen, 1998). Developmental research on metacognition (Flammer, 1995) suggests that children, especially in the preschool period, either grossly overestimate their capacities or underestimate tasks and only during the middle elementary school years do they become more realistic. Thus where individuals differ in their cognitive development, self-efficacy scores obtained with children aged 8-12 are to some degree biased in the sense of overestimating their diabetes management capacities and underestimating the recommended diabetes self-care tasks.

In the life of adolescents other developmental issues play an important role. This age group is in the transition from being dependent children to becoming independent adults. Adolescence is a period of discovering one's identity and one's sexuality, attending school, and making friends. In diabetes management these present challenges and affect the person's appraisal of self-efficacy (Grey, Kanner, & Lacey, 1999).

Adults and older adults are confronted with other issues like work, raising children, and retirement. These aspects of a person's life also affect daily diabetes management behaviors. Finally, old age clearly brings decreasing capacities, with consequences for a self-efficacy scale.

## Instrument Format and Terminology Issues

The traditional measurement of self-efficacy requires that individuals rate their degree of confidence in performing a specific task on a 0 to 10 or 0 to 100 semantically anchored scale (0 = cannot do at all, and 10 or 100 = highly confident). Seven- or 5-point scales have also been used (e.g., 1 = not at all sure to 5 or 7 = completely sure) (Maibach & Murphy, 1995).

In our development and testing of the Dutch diabetes management self-efficacy instrument for people with type 2 diabetes, a simple 5-point rating scale was found a usable format (van der Bijl et al., 1999). Since this rating scale differed from the English version of the scale used in the United States and a different format was recommended by the panel of experts, a study was conducted to see how closely the different terminologies and formats (see Figure 2.3) were correlated (Shortridge-Baggett & van der Bijl, 1996). The correlation coefficients ranged from $r = 0.92$ for Format "A" with Format "D" to $r = 0.99$ for Format "B" with Format "C." Since all correlations were acceptable, any format can be used. The recommended formats are "B" and "C."

In general, items and the response scale should be presented at the reading level of the respondents (Bandura, 1997b). For individuals with lower literacy skills, including children, alternative forms of data collection should be considered. In a recent study investigating the variables influencing self-efficacy, the researcher has chosen to use the scales as structured interviews (Lintel Hekkert, 2000). With interviews nonresponses due to respondents' inability to fill out paper and pencil instruments can be prevented. With the self-efficacy scale for children with diabetes two symbolic response scales were tested: for example, faces and thumbs (Kappen, 1998). Both symbols have been interpreted in the same way. Bandura (1997b), however, recommends not using happy or sad faces for children, with the argument that young children may misread the scale as measuring happiness or sadness rather than how confident they are that they can perform given tasks. The created rating scale with hands with a thumb up ranging from small to big is a useful alternative for the response scale with the faces. The thumb up symbol is in our opinion a perfect pictorial descriptor of confidence, because it represents the meaning of "Okay, I can do it." Moreover, the use of thumbs with progressively larger size also has the advantage that the size gradations represent increasing confidence that children can perform the tasks. Therefore, we recommend rating

## Format A

1. I think I'm able to check my blood sugar if necessary:
  ☐ yes, definitely
  ☐ probably yes
  ☐ maybe yes, maybe no
  ☐ probably no
  ☐ no, definitely not

2. I think I'm able to select the right foods:
  ☐ yes, definitely
  ☐ probably yes
  ☐ maybe yes, maybe no
  ☐ probably no
  ☐ no, definitely not

3. I think I'm able to adjust my diet when I'm ill:
  ☐ yes, definitely

*continued* ... ... ....

## Format B

| | Yes Definitely | Probably Yes | Maybe Yes Maybe No | Probably No | Definitely Not |
|---|---|---|---|---|---|
| 1. I think I'm able to check my blood sugar | ☐ | ☐ | ☐ | ☐ | ☐ |
| 2. I think I'm able to select the right foods | ☐ | ☐ | ☐ | ☐ | ☐ |
| 3. I think I'm able to adjust my diet when I'm ill | ☐ | ☐ | ☐ | ☐ | ☐ |

*continued* ... ... ....

## Format C

**CONFIDENCE**

       A        B        C        D        E
Very little  + —————— + —————— + —————— + —————— +  Very much

How much confidence do you have in:
1. Checking your blood sugar    A  B  C  D  E
2. Selecting the right foods    A  B  C  D  E
3. Adjusting your diet when you're ill    A  B  C  D  E

*continued* ... ... ....

## Format D

**CONFIDENCE**

    A        B        C        D        E
Very little  + —————— + —————— + —————— + —————— +  Very much

                        How much confidence do you have in:
A  B  C  D  E    1. Checking your blood sugar
A  B  C  D  E    2. Selecting the right foods
A  B  C  D  E    3. Adjusting your diet when you're ill

*continued* ... ... ....

**Figure 2.3.** Different formats and terminology for self-efficacy instruments (Shortridge-Baggett & van der Bijl, 1996).

scales with thumbs up instead of rating scales with faces in the measurement of self-efficacy in young children.

## SUMMARY OF METHODOLOGICAL ISSUES

We have seen that in operationalizing the concept of self-efficacy, the most important point is that self-efficacy scales must be tailored to specific domains of functioning. Thus, self-efficacy instruments should be named for the behavioral domain they represent. Self-efficacy is related to the specific behaviors and contexts in which it occurs. Even within the well defined domain of diabetes management, the complexity of behaviors and situational contexts vary from population to population, depending on the type of diabetes and age. Therefore, in developing any self-efficacy scale, and in establishing the content validity of the scale, individual or focus group interviews with members of the target population are needed to identify the most relevant tasks and the corresponding competencies, barriers and challenges. The self-efficacy dimensions of strength, magnitude, and generality should be part of a self-efficacy scale in order to have valid self-efficacy items across a variety of tasks and linked to difficult situations within the behavioral domains of interest.

## REFERENCES

Bandura, A. (1977). Self-efficacy: Toward a unifying theory of behavioral change. *Psychological Review, 84*, 191-215.

Bandura, A. (1986). *Social foundations of thought and action: A social cognitive theory.* Englewoods Cliffs, NJ: Prentice Hall.

Bandura, A. (Ed.). (1995). *Self-efficacy in changing societies.* New York: Press Syndicate of the University of Cambridge.

Bandura, A. (1997a). *Self-efficacy: The exercise of control.* New York: Freeman.

Bandura, A. (1997b). *Guide for constructing self-efficacy scales.* Unpublished guide. Stanford University, Stanford, CA.

Bandura, A., & Cervone, D. (1983). Self-evaluative and self-efficacy mechanisms governing the motivational effects of goal systems. *Journal of Personality and Social Psychology, 45*, 1017-1028.

Bijl, J. van der, Poelgeest-Eeltink, A. van, & Shortridge-Baggett, L. (1999). The psychometric properties of the diabetes management self-efficacy scale for patients with Type 2 diabetes Mellitus. *Journal of Advanced Nursing, 30*(2), 352-359.

Coppel, D. B. (1980). *Relationship of perceived social support and self-efficacy to major and minor stresses.* Unpublished doctoral dissertation, University of Washington, Seattle.

DiIorio, C., Faherty, B., & Manteuffel, B. (1994). Epilepsy self-management: Partial replication and extension. *Research in Nursing and Health, 17*, 167-174.

Flammer, A. (1995). Development analysis on control beliefs. In A. Bandura (Ed.), *Self-efficacy in changing societies.* New York: Press Syndicate of the University of Cambridge.

Geest, S. de (1996). *Subclinical noncompliance with immunosuppressive therapy in heart transplant recipients: A cluster analytic study.* Doctoral dissertation, Leuven, University of Leuven, Netherlands.

Gist, M. E., & Mitchell, T. R. (1992). Self-efficacy: A theoretical analysis of its determinants and malleability. *Academy of Management Review, 17,* 2, 183-206.

Grey, M., Kanner, S., & Lacey, K. O. (1999). Characteristics of the learner: Children and adolescents. *Diabetes Educator, 25*(Suppl. 6), 25-33.

Grey, M., Boland, E. A., Davidson, M., Yu, C., & Tamborlane, W. V. (1999). Coping skills training for youths with diabetes on intensive therapy. *Applied Nursing Research, 12*(1), 3-12.

Hockmeyer, M. T. (1990). *The influence of self-efficacy and health beliefs, considering treatment mode, on self-care behavior of adults diagnosed within 3 years with non-insulin-dependent diabetes mellitus.* Doctoral dissertation, University of Maryland, Baltimore.

Kappen, M. J. (1998). *Het ontwikkelen van een meetinstrument dat bij kinderen van 8-12 jaar met insuline-afhankelijke diabetes mellitus self-efficacy beliefs meet ten aanzien van hun diabetes zelfzorg* [Instrument development and testing for self-efficacy beliefs in diabetes management of children 8 to 12 years of age with insulin dependent diabetes mellitus]. Master's thesis, Division of Nursing Science, University of Utrecht in collaboration with the University of Maastricht, the Netherlands.

Kavanagh, D. J., & Bower, G. H. (1985). Mood and self-efficacy: Impact of joy and sadness on perceived capabilities. *Cognitive Therapy and Research, 9,* 507-525.

Lintel Hekkert, M. (2000). *De invloed van psycho-sociale factoren op self-efficacy bij patiënten met niet-insuline-afhankelijke diabetes mellitus* [The influence of psychosocial factors on self-efficacy with noninsulin-dependent patients with diabetes mellitus]. Master's thesis, Division of Nursing Science, University of Utrecht in collaboration with the University of Maastricht, the Netherlands.

Maibach, E., & Murphy, D. A. (1995). Self-efficacy in health promotion research and practice: Conceptualization and measurement. *Health Education Research, 10*(1), 37-50.

Meyaard, T. (1996). Workshop "Diabetes mellitus en migranten" [Workshop "Diabetes mellitus and migrants"]. *EADE Nieuwsbrief, 11*(2), 47-49.

Moens, A. (1998). *Ontwikkeling van een valide en betrouwbaar meetinstrument dat perceived self-efficacy meet ten aanzien van diabetes zelfzorg bij adolescenten met Type 1 diabetes mellitus* [Development of a valid and reliable measuring instrument, measuring diabetes self-care perceived self-efficacy with adolescents with Type 1 diabetes mellitus]. Master's thesis, University of Gent, Belgium.

Pajares, F. (1997). Current directions in self-efficacy research. In M. Maehr & P. R. Pintrich (Eds.), *Advances in motivation and achievement* (Vol. 10, pp. 1-49). Greenwich, CT: JAI Press.

Peltenburg, L. (1995). Wat is diabetes? [What is diabetes?]. In A. L. Peltenburg, K. M. J. Krans, H. E. A. Dassen, R. J. Heine, & E. Van Ballegooie (Eds.), Diabetes mellitus. Cahiers Bio-wetenschappen en Maatschappij (17e jaargang, nr. 4). Stichting biowetenschappen en maatschappij, Utrecht, the Netherlands.

Schaalma, H. (1993). De analyse van gedragsdeterminanten [The analysis of the determinants of behavior]. In V. Damoiseaux, H. T. van der Molen, & G. J. Kok (Eds.), *Gezondheidsvoorlichting en gedragsverandering.* Assen, the Netherlands: Van Gorcum.

Schneewind, K. A. (1995). Impact of family processes on control beliefs. In Bandura, A. (Ed.), *Self-efficacy in changing societies.* New York: Press Syndicate of the University of Cambridge.

Schunk, D. H., & Carbonari, J. (1984). Self-efficacy models. In J. Matarazzo, S. Weiss, J. Herd, N. Miller, & S. Weiss (Eds.), *Behavioral health: A handbook of health enhancement and disease prevention.* New York: John Wiley & Sons.

Schwarzer, R. (1993). *Measurement of perceived self-efficacy: Psychometric scales for cross-cultural research.* Berlin: Freie Universität Berlin, Institut für Psychologie.

Shortridge-Baggett, L. M., & Bijl, J. J. van der (1996). International collaborative research on management self-efficacy in diabetes mellitus. *The Journal of the New York State Nurses Association, 27*(3), 9-14.

Smith, M. S., Wallston, K. A., & Smith, C. A. (1995). The development and validation of the Perceived Health Competence Scale. *Health Education Research, 10*(1), 51-64.

Strecher, V., DeVellis, B. M., Becker, M. H., & Rosenstock, I. M. (1986). The role of self-efficacy in achieving health behavior change. *Health Education Quarterly, 13,* 73-91.

Taal, E. (1995). *Self-efficacy, self-management and patient education in rheumatoid arthritis.* Doctoral dissertation, University of Twente, Enschede, the Netherlands.

Talbot, F., Nouwen, A., Gringas, J., Gosselin, M., & Audet, J. (1997). The assessment of diabetes-related cognitive and social factors: The multidimensional diabetes questionnaire. *Journal of Behavioral Medicine, 20*(3), 291-312.

Weiner, B. (1979). A theory of motivation for some classroom experiences. *Journal of Educational Psychology, 71,* 3-25.

Weiner, B. (1985). An attributional theory of achievement, motivation and emotion. *Psychological Review, 92,* 548-573.

## APPENDIX

Directions:
Please answer each question by checking the answer that describes how convinced you are in managing your diabetes.

|  | Yes Definitely | Probably Yes | Maybe Yes Maybe No | Probably No | Definitely Not |
|---|---|---|---|---|---|
| 1. I think I'm able to check my blood sugar if necessary. | ❑ | ❑ | ❑ | ❑ | ❑ |
| 2. I think I'm able to correct my blood sugar when the blood sugar value is too high. | ❑ | ❑ | ❑ | ❑ | ❑ |
| 3. I think I'm able to correct my blood sugar when the blood sugar value is too low. | ❑ | ❑ | ❑ | ❑ | ❑ |
| 4. I think I'm able to select the right foods. | ❑ | ❑ | ❑ | ❑ | ❑ |
| 5. I think I'm able to select different foods but stay within my diabetic diet. | ❑ | ❑ | ❑ | ❑ | ❑ |
| 6. I think I'm able to keep my weight under control. | ❑ | ❑ | ❑ | ❑ | ❑ |
| 7. I think I'm able to examine my feet for skin problems. | ❑ | ❑ | ❑ | ❑ | ❑ |
| 8. I think I'm able to get sufficient physical activities, for example, taking a walk or biking. | ❑ | ❑ | ❑ | ❑ | ❑ |
| 9. I think I'm able to adjust my diet when I'm ill. | ❑ | ❑ | ❑ | ❑ | ❑ |
| 10. I think I'm able to follow my diet most of the time. | ❑ | ❑ | ❑ | ❑ | ❑ |
| 11. I think I'm able to take extra physical activities, when the doctor advises me to do so. | ❑ | ❑ | ❑ | ❑ | ❑ |
| 12. When taking extra physical activities, I think I'm able to adjust my diet. | ❑ | ❑ | ❑ | ❑ | ❑ |

| | Yes Definitely | Probably Yes | Maybe Yes Maybe No | Probably No | Definitely Not |
|---|---|---|---|---|---|
| 13. I think I'm able to follow my diet when I am away from home. | ❑ | ❑ | ❑ | ❑ | ❑ |
| 14. I think I'm able to adjust my diet when I am away from home. | ❑ | ❑ | ❑ | ❑ | ❑ |
| 15. I think I'm able to follow my diet when I am on vacation. | ❑ | ❑ | ❑ | ❑ | ❑ |
| 16. I think I'm able to follow my diet when I am at a reception/party. | ❑ | ❑ | ❑ | ❑ | ❑ |
| 17. I think I'm able to adjust my diet when I am under stress or tension. | ❑ | ❑ | ❑ | ❑ | ❑ |
| 18. I think I'm able to visit the doctor once a year to monitor my diabetes. | ❑ | ❑ | ❑ | ❑ | ❑ |

Would you please answer the next two questions if you take medication (pills) for your diabetes. If you do not take medication to control your diabetes, you can skip these two questions and continue with the general questions.

| | Yes Definitely | Probably Yes | Maybe Yes Maybe No | Probably No | Definitely Not |
|---|---|---|---|---|---|
| 19. I think I'm able to take my medicine as prescribed. | ❑ | ❑ | ❑ | ❑ | ❑ |
| 20. I think I'm able to adjust my medication when I'm ill. | ❑ | ❑ | ❑ | ❑ | ❑ |

*Note.* The *Diabetes Management Self-Efficacy Scale for Type 2 Diabetes* is developed by the University of Utrecht, division of Nursing Science, P.O. Box 85060, 3508 AB Utrecht, The Netherlands.

# Part II
# Self-Efficacy in Diabetes Management

# 3

# Self-Efficacy in Children With Diabetes Mellitus: Testing of a Measurement Instrument

Michel J. Kappen
Jaap J. van der Bijl
Mary Joan Vaccaro-Olko

Diabetes mellitus is a chronic metabolic disorder, involving a defect in insulin production, insulin action or both, and resulting in hyperglycemia. Type 1 diabetes results from a cell-mediated autoimmune process which leads to complete destruction of the beta cells of the pancreas and an absolute deficiency of insulin production. Exogenous insulin by injection or continuous insulin pump therapy is required for glucose homeostasis. In type 2 diabetes, the defect in insulin production stems from both insulin resistance and a relative insulin deficiency, or a primary insulin secretory defect with insulin resistance. This type of diabetes usually afflicts people who are sedentary, obese and older and is initially managed by diet, exercise, and weight reduction, though oral hypoglycemic agents are also commonly required to achieve glycemic control. Type 1 diabetes represents 10%-15% of cases, while the more prevalent form of diabetes, type 2, accounts for 85%-90%.

In diabetes mellitus, self-management is critical for preventing complications but difficult for all; it is even more challenging for children and their families. In order to ensure an acceptable blood glucose level, children and their parents need to master a complex set of diabetes self-management tasks, and most of the tasks need to be executed daily. The diabetes nurse specialist plays a central role in teaching knowledge and skills to children with diabetes and their parents. Research on the effect of diabetes education, however, has revealed that knowledge and skills have limited effects on actual diabetes self-management behaviors (Kaplan et al., 1985; Padgett et al., 1988; Pennings-van der Eerden, 1992). Clearly interventions that focus on behavior change are needed to obtain better effects.

According to Bandura (1982,1986,1992), self-efficacy, or people's judgments about their ability to organize and execute courses of action to attain desired outcomes, determines whether or not knowledge and skills are actually employed to successfully execute the courses of action. Thus self-efficacy may be a key element in successful self-management behavior. A number of studies have found that self-efficacy was a major predictor of successful diabetes self-management. These studies, however, used samples of adults with diabetes and data from the studies cannot be used to determine the predictive value of self-efficacy in children with diabetes (Kappen, 1995). A clearer understanding of self-efficacy in children requires additional research, which in turn requires valid and reliable instruments for measuring self-efficacy in children.

If children are to be reliable and accurate reporters of self-efficacy, a measurement instrument must be tailored to their developmental level (LaGreca, 1990; Reynolds, 1993). A child needs both the general skills to complete an instrument and the ability to self-perceive, since self-efficacy is a kind of self-perception (Flammer, 1995). As for general skills, in order to complete an instrument, a child needs to have sufficient reading skills and an idea of grammar. The minimal age for those skills is 7 years, after 1 year of primary school on average (LaGreca, 1990; Reynolds, 1993). The language of the instrument needs to be tailored as much as possible to the level of reading and understanding of the child. Supporting the text with images or symbols is also suggested (Reynolds, 1993).

Development of the concept of capability runs more or less parallel to development of children in the way they perceive the world around them. During the first years of primary school children describe others mainly in terms of concrete physical characteristics like their looks ("Ann has brown eyes"), possessions ("Marc has got a bike"), or specific behaviors ("Mandy hits me"). They are not yet able to perceive more abstract properties like thoughts and feelings. This ability begins to develop at about 8 years of age and matures fully only in adolescence (Stone & Lemanek, 1990). Thus children at 7 years of age do not distinguish between natural ability and effort. They think that hard workers are automatically clever. In addition, they are not familiar with the concept of task-difficulty. During primary school they begin to differentiate capability into natural ability, effort, task difficulty, and luck. During primary school achievements of children at school start to count and feedback by way of marks makes it clear that there are differences between children and that achievements depend not on effort alone (Flammer, 1995; Stone & Lemanek, 1990).

The ability to make a judgment about one's own capability does not develop in all areas at the same time. It is first attained in domains in which children acquire much experience, such as school achievements (Flammer, 1995). Because from the moment they are confronted with diabetes mellitus, children have a role in its management, this might also be considered an area of experience.

Children often experience their capability as not stable, so their perception of it can change from day to day (Stone & Lemanek, 1990). In addition, younger children tend to overestimate their capability or underestimate the difficulty of a task. They also regard their effort as inexhaustible. In other words, with sufficient effort everything is achievable. During elementary school such perceptions are modified to become more realistic because of the ongoing feedback children receive (Flammer, 1995).

The study reported here was designed to create a valid and reliable Dutch instrument to measure diabetes management self-efficacy in children ages 8 to 12 taking into account this developmental trajectory.

# METHODS

## Instrument Development

*Content Validity.* Instrument development and assessment of content validity were based on the procedures recommended by Lynn (1986). The Children's Management Self-Efficacy of Diabetes (CMSED) scale (Shortridge-Baggett & Roden, 1994), a comparable instrument developed for children with diabetes in the United States, did not use the Lynn procedures for establishing content validity and several items focused more on knowledge than behavior. Therefore, that scale was examined but not completely followed. In order to measure self-efficacy about specific tasks, a 23-item list was compiled from the literature on self-management activities relevant for children with diabetes. The list was then examined by a panel of nine diabetes specialist nurses for relevance (Lynn, 1986). Eight of the experts were employed at outpatient clinics of general and teaching hospitals in the western part of The Netherlands. One expert was employed in a medical orthopedagogical institute for children with diabetes in the middle of the country.

The experts received a brief explanation of both the study and the concept to be measured and they were asked to score the items with regard to relevance on a 4-point ordinal scale, in which:

1 = not relevant
2 = unable to assess relevance without item revision
3 = relevant but needs minor alteration
4 = very relevant and succinct.

Using this rating scale made it possible not only to quantify the content validity of the individual items, but also to determine the Content Validity Index (CVI) for the instrument as a whole. The CVI is the number of items judged relevant (score of 3 or 4) in proportion to the total number of items (Lynn, 1986). The advantage of quantifying the relevance of the items is that they can be dropped or selected based on a "solid" score. The experts were consulted in two rounds.

*Development of an Appropriate Rating Scale.* In the study of Shortridge-Baggett and van der Bijl (1996) good results were obtained in measurement of self-efficacy in adults with type 2 diabetes, using a 5-point Likert scale. This scale contained the following rating categories:

• yes certainly
• probably yes
• maybe yes/maybe no

- probably not
- certainly not

After reviewing the literature on using self-report in children (Flanery, 1990; Reynolds, 1993) and consultation with an expert in this area, however, it became clear that the scale needed to be adapted to the developmental level of children. The phrases probably yes and probably not would be too abstract for children, so these were changed into a little certain yes and a little certain no (the closest translation for the original Dutch wording). In addition, instructions that would be clear and comprehensible for children were added to the instrument, for example "If you are certain that you can not do it, then put a mark in box 1."

Since a scale becomes more understandable for young children if it is supported with images/symbols, two kinds of symbols were tested:

1. First, a scale using faces with an expression varying from sad/gloomy to glad/gay was developed. Faces are frequently used and are effective symbols for self-report in children. Bandura (1997), however, has advised against happy or sad faces to measure self-efficacy, because children may misread the scale as measuring their happiness or sadness rather than their confidence in performing tasks.
2. A rating scale using hands with a thumb up, ranging from small to big, was also created (see Figure 3.1). The idea was that a thumb up (symbol of "Okay, you can do it") is an adequate pictorial descriptor of confidence and also that thumbs with progressively larger sizes could be used with the explanation that the size gradations represented increasing confidence that the child could perform the tasks.

To test these two versions, 10 self-efficacy questions were formulated with both rating scales (faces and thumbs) on the topics of swimming and gymnastics. Next, the scales were submitted to eight children between 8 and 12 years old. The criteria used for judging the scales were understandability/clarity, potential to differentiate between the rating categories, and the preference of the child. The test results of both the rating scales are described in the Results section of this article.

***Clarity.*** In order to assess the clarity and understandability of the instrument for children with diabetes, a pretest was conducted in a children's hospital. The item

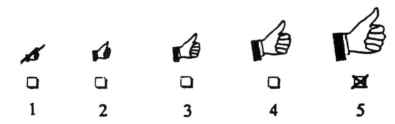

**Figure 3.1.** Example of the "thumb up" rating scale (Kappen, 1998).

list was submitted to four children; two were 8 years of age, one was 10, and one was 12. The children were asked to complete the instrument aloud so that we could hear possible difficulties. Next, the following questions were asked, based in part on a questionnaire developed by Thibodeau and Hawkins (1989), to assess the face validity of an instrument:

- Do you have problems understanding the question?
- Are the words clear to you?

The children were also asked:

- Are the instructions clear? Can you tell what you are asked to do?
- Are there questions that you would rather not answer?

In addition, attention was given to the nonverbal reactions of the child as cues that something was unclear to the child. For all the children, the instructions for the instrument appeared clear and understandable and most of the items could be read by them. A few items were a problem for the two 8-year-old children, because they contained difficult words. Therefore a few minor alterations were made.

## Instrument Testing

***Sample Selection.*** The diabetes teams of three hospitals in the western part of The Netherlands were asked to participate in instrument testing. Two of the hospitals were specialized children's hospitals. All three teams agreed to participate and the Institutional Review Boards approved the proposal.

Participants were selected by reviewing the schedules of outpatient clinics for children who had an appointment during the next week(s). The diabetes nurse checked to determine whether participation of a child was contraindicated for psychosocial reasons. The children were selected and their parents received a letter which described the study, asked them to participate, indicated that personal data and answers would be confidential, and assured them that participation was voluntary and not related to the treatment of the child. When the children and their parents arrived at the outpatient clinic, they were asked if they were willing to participate. When they agreed, the child and one of the parents signed an informed consent form.

***Reliability Testing.*** To test the reliability of the instrument (Clark & Watson, 1995), the score distributions of individual items were examined. Then, internal consistency of the instrument was examined by determination of Cronbach's alpha and analysis of interitem correlations.

***Criterion-Related Validity Testing.*** Evidence of criterion-related validity was sought by determining whether self-efficacy was a predictive factor in the diabetes self-management behaviors of children. The total scores of children on the instrument were used. Diabetes self-management was operationalized by HbA1c measurement and the opinion of the diabetes nurse about the actual performance of children of diabetes self-management behaviors.

"Glycohemoglobin (GHb), also commonly referred to as glycated hemoglobin, glycosylated hemoglobin, HbA1c or HbA1, is used to describe a series of stable minor hemoglobin components formed slowly and nonenzymatically from hemoglobin and glucose" (Goldstein & Little, 1997, p. 481). The normal range for GHb is 4% to 7% (Goldstein & Little, 1997). Glycohemoglobin is formed through a nonenzymatic interaction between glucose and the amino groups of the valine and lysine residues in hemoglobin (Colman et al., 1997). The speed of formation of GHb is related directly to blood glucose concentration. Since the average erythrocyte is freely permeable to glucose and has a life of 120 days, the GHb in a blood sample provides a history of glycemic control for the previous 2 to 3 months. Caloric intake, insulin and exercise do not influence HbA1c. This test can be performed at any time of day. Therefore, HbA1c is a good objective measurement of glycemic control of diabetes mellitus over time.

Four principal techniques are used to measure glycohemoglobin: ion-exchange chromatography, electrophoresis, affinity chromatography and immunoassay. Each assay measures slightly different glycated products. At present, comparison of the results from two different laboratories is not possible.

A blood sample was obtained from each child in this study to measure HbA1c. The three hospital laboratories involved appeared to use the same method for determining HbA1c and normal measures were nearly identical, suggesting that the measures collected did not need to be recalculated to be compared. In the outpatient clinics the HbA1c of the children was tested once every 2 to 3 months. The absolute HbA1c values were not used for feedback to children and parents. A categorization was used instead. For correlations with self-efficacy scores, therefore, comparable categories of HbA1c were used in this study. Table 3.1 outlines the categorizations.

HbA1c measures provide an image of glycemic control in the period preceding the test. According to Bandura (1982, 1986), however, self-efficacy influences behavior that remains to be executed. Using HbA1c measures, therefore, assumes

**Table 3.1.** Categories of HbA1c values (SKZ, 1994).

| Hospital | | This study | |
|---|---|---|---|
| < 6.3% | no diabetes | | |
| 6.3% - 7.0% | sharp | | |
| 7.1% - 9.0% | good | 9.0 % | good |
| 9.1% - 10.0% | moderate | 9.1% - 10.0% | moderate |
| 10.1% - 12.0% | bad | > 10.0% | bad |
| > 12.0% | hospital admission required | | |

that the self-efficacy of children at the time of completing the instrument did not differ from that in the preceding period. For assessing criterion-related validity of the instrument, our expectation was that the higher the self-efficacy total score, the better the diabetes self-management and thus the lower the HbA1c measure. In addition to the HbA1c measure taken on the day of participation in the study, the mean of the last three tests was used to prevent possible fluctuations.

To assess self-management by the children, the diabetes nurse was asked "What is your opinion of the actual performance of diabetes self-management activities by the child?" A 5-point Likert scale was used with the categories of bad, moderate, sufficient, quite good, good. Because the opinion of the nurse was based on the preceding period, the assessment of construct validity assumed that self-efficacy would be reasonably constant in children. We expected that the higher the self-efficacy total score, the higher the nurse's opinion score would be.

## RESULTS

### Instrument Development

*Content Validity.* In the first expert round concerning the 23-item list all nine experts completed the score form, for a 100% response rate. All 23 items were found to be content valid by the experts, based upon the decision rule of Lynn (1986) that an item, in order to be called content valid when consulting nine experts, must receive a score of 3 or 4 on the rating scale by at least seven of the experts. Because all items were judged content valid, the content validity index (CVI) for the entire item-list reached the maximum score of 1. After the first round, therefore, the instrument could be regarded as content valid.

The experts provided several suggestions for changing the content of the items. In some items the phrasing was changed; a few items were added; a few items were combined into one item; the sequence of the item clusters was altered; the clusters were provided with "leaders"; and finally, for four items an introductory, context-describing sentence was added. These alterations resulted in a new list of 29 items.

In the second expert round, the response rate was lower. Seven out of nine experts (78%) completed the score form. Again, for all 29 items the scores were sufficient to be called content valid (a score of 3 or 4 by a minimum of six experts [Lynn, 1986]) The CVI of the entire list again reached the maximum value of 1.

This version of the instrument could, therefore, also be called content valid. Still, based on some suggestions of the experts, a few minor alterations were made in the wording of some items. In addition, an item that was dropped after the first round, although having a good score, was reincluded, making a total of 30 items. These alterations did not necessitate another expert review.

*Rating Scale.* The tests of the two rating scales did not show differences in clarity, understandability and potential to differentiate. The preferences of the children differed, however. The younger children preferred the scale with the faces, while most older children preferred the scale with the hands. With only these minor differences, the choice was made to use the scale with the hands, because in our opinion this symbol is the best representation of self-efficacy and the dimension of strength.

## Instrument Testing

*Sample.* The sample available for assessing reliability and construct validity consisted of 30 children, 11 boys and 19 girls. The ages of the children varied from 8 to 12 years with a mean of 10.3 and a standard deviation of 1.2 years. The number of years a child had had diabetes varied from 0.33 to 10.00 with a mean of 4.63 and a standard deviation of 2.98 years. The distribution of the sample over the three hospitals was 14, 13 and 3 children.

*Reliability.* Nine items were scored extremely high; that is, on these items almost all respondents (90% or more) gave the same answer, a score of 5. Other scores were chosen only sporadically, and the score of 4 prevailed. Eleven items showed a little more variation, but still a score of 5 was preponderant. On 10 items, the scores were distributed more equally, though still with a relatively small representation of lower scores. The mean score for 28 items was 4 or higher. The mean scores for the other two items were 3.3 and 3.7. Cronbach's alpha for the instrument was calculated at 0.71. This is a sufficient value for comparing groups of respondents (Polit & Hungler, 1999). Because the instrument was internally consistent, a factor analysis was of interest. Factor analysis, however, was not possible since the recommended number of respondents required for this analysis was 200 to 300 (Comrey, 1988), several times the size of the study sample.

The mean interitem correlation was 0.11. The lowest correlation was -0.27 and the highest 1.00. Thus there were big differences in interitem correlations. The value of 1.00 can be explained by the fact that two items received a score of 5 from all respondents. These data indicate that the instrument was not homogeneous.

*Criterion-Related Validity.* The results of the criterion-related validity assessment of the instrument are shown in Table 3.2. The correlation of the self-efficacy total score with the HbA1c measure on the day of the study (SE total—HbA1c) and the correlation of the mean self-efficacy total score with the mean HbA1c measure

**Table 3.2.** Correlations for criterion-related validity assessment.

| 1. SE total – HbA1c | $\rho$ (Spearman) = - 0.21 (p = 0.44) |
|---|---|
| 2. SE total – HbA1c mean | $\rho$ (Spearman) = - 0.12 (p = 0.60) |
| 3. SE total – Opinion nurse | r (Pearson)   =   0.23 (p = 0.24) |

(SE total—HbA1c mean) are noted, along with the correlation between the self-efficacy total scores of the children and the opinion of the diabetes specialist nurse on their performance of their diabetes self-management tasks. No significant relationships were found. Therefore, criterion-validity of the instrument was not supported.

## DISCUSSION

The instrument seemed promising in the developmental stage and it was judged content valid by experts. The instructions and the items of the instrument were clear and comprehensible for children. In addition, a rating scale was developed and tested using symbols that were found to be adequate and attractive for children.

Based upon these results, satisfying results were expected in the main study. The results of the test of the instrument, however, were disappointing. The most striking finding was the limited variation in the item scores. A considerable number of items were scored high by all the children. Therefore, the instrument did not distinguish between children in regard to self-efficacy. Assuming that the rating scale functioned well, this "ceiling effect" indicates that the items described tasks that were too easy for children in the sample or that were interpreted as such.

One explanation for the ceiling effect may be the sample itself. The majority of the children had had experience with diabetes self-management for a number of years, though the instrument was developed primarily for newly diagnosed children. Also, Bandura (1984) states that people make self-efficacy judgments about tasks and situations with which they feel uncertain or unfamiliar. The concept is more concerned with courses of action than with trivial individual actions. Bandura illustrates this with the example of driving a car. Turning the ignition key, moving the gear-stick, watching traffic signs and such are trivial motor skills and therefore not relevant. What is relevant is the overall capability to maneuver a car and handle traffic situations in circumstances that vary in difficulty (in daytime or at night, on a lonely country road or crowded city traffic and so on). Some of the items in our instrument contained more or less "trivial actions."

For this instrument items were derived from a literature review, interviews with diabetes specialist nurses, and an instrument developed in the United States. Maibach and Murphy (1995), however, consider interviews with representatives from the target population the best source for obtaining relevant items on self-efficacy. They also note that self-efficacy varies with circumstances and situations. For an adequate measurement of self-efficacy, the items on an instrument should vary according to the difficulty of the situation. Not varying the items weakens the predictive power of the instrument. The instrument developed in this study did not fully meet these criteria. Consideration should be given to this in further instrument development.

Given the limited variance in the scores on the self-efficacy items, the lack of support for the criterion-related validity of the instrument is not surprising. In addition, the use of HbA1c as an indicator of diabetes self-management behavior might be problematic. The relationship between self-efficacy and diabetes self-management in general is reported to be stronger than the relationship of self-management behavior and HbA1c (Kavanagh et al., 1993; McCaul et al., 1987). Besides, other factors influence HbA1c, such as individual differences in psychophysiological reactions to stress and genetic constitution (Jacobson et al., 1990). Finally, children with diabetes share their responsibility for regulation with their parents. Depending on their age, diabetes management is more or less structured by the parents.

Self-efficacy has been shown to be an important concept in diabetes education. This initial self-efficacy measurement instrument in the Dutch language for children with diabetes mellitus can be used for clinical assessments to guide teaching about daily diabetes self-management tasks to be performed by the newly diagnosed child. Further development and testing of the scale is needed, however, especially for children more experienced with diabetes mellitus.

## REFERENCES

American Diabetes Association. (2000). Clinical practice recommendations 2000. *Diabetes Care, 23*(1), S4-S19.

Bandura, A. (1977). Self-efficacy: Toward a unifying theory of behavior change. *Psychological Review, 84*(2), 191-212.

Bandura, A. (1982). Self-efficacy mechanism in human agency. *American Psychologist, 37*(2), 122-147.

Bandura, A. (1984). Recycling misconceptions of perceived self-efficacy. *Cognitive Therapy and Research, 8*(3), 231-255.

Bandura, A. (1986). *Social foundation of thought and action: A social cognitive theory.* Englewood Cliffs, NJ: Prentice Hall.

Bandura, A. (1991). Social cognitive theory of self-regulation. *Organizational Behavior and Human Decision Processes, 50,* 248-287.

Bandura, A. (1992). Exercise of personal agency through the self-efficacy mechanism. In R. Schwarzer (Ed.), *Self-efficacy: Thought control of action* (pp. 30-38). Washington, DC: Hemisphere Publishing Corporation.

Bandura, A. (1995). Exercise of personal and collective efficacy in changing societies. In A. Bandura (Ed.), *Self-efficacy in changing societies* (pp. 1-45). New York: Press Syndicate of the University of Cambridge.

Bandura, A. (1997). *Guide for constructing self-efficacy scales.* Unpublished guide. Stanford University.

Clark, L. A., & Watson, D. (1995). Constructing validity: Basic issues in objective scale development. *Psychological assessment, 7*(3), 309-319.

Colman, P. G., Goodall, G. I., Garcia-Webb, P., Williams, P. F., & Dunlop, M. E. (1997). *Glycohaemoglobin: A crucial measurement in modern diabetes management: Progress towards standardization and improved precision of measurement.* Australian Diabetes Society, the Royal College of Pathologists of Australasia and the Australasian Association of Clinical Biochemist Consensus Conference.

Comrey, A. L. (1988). Factor-analytic methods of scale development in personality and clinical psychology. *Journal of Consulting and Clinical Psychology, 56,* 754-761.

De Heus, P., van der Leeden, R., & Gazendam, B. (1995). *Toegepaste data-analyse: Technieken voor niet-experimenteel onderzoek in de sociale wetenschappen* [Applied data-analysis: Techniques for non-experimental research in the social sciences]. Utrecht: Lemma BV.

Flammer, A. (1995). Developmental analysis on control beliefs. In A. Bandura (Ed.), *Self-efficacy in changing societies* (pp. 69-113). New York: Press Syndicate of the University of Cambridge.

Flanery, R. C. (1990). Methodological and psychometric considerations in child reports. In A. M. LaGreca (Ed.), *Through the eyes of the child: Obtaining self-reports from children and adolescents* (pp. 3-17). Boston: Allyn and Bacon.

Goldstein, D. E., Little, R. R., Lorenz, R. A., Malone, J. I., Nathan, D., & Peterson, C. M. (1995). Tests of glycemia in diabetes. *Diabetes Care, 18*(6), 896-909.

Goldstein, D. E., & Little, R. R. (1997). Monitoring glycemia in diabetes. *Endocrinology and Metabolism Clinics of North America, 26*(3), 475-486.

Grey, M., Kanner, S., & Lacey, K. O. (1999). Characteristics of the learner: Children and adolescents. *The Diabetes Educator, 25*(6), 25-33.

Jacobson, A. M., Adler, A. G., Wolsdorf, J. L., Anderson, B., & Derby, L. (1990). Psychological characteristics of adults with IDDM. *Diabetes Care, 13,* 375-381.

Kaplan, R. M., Chadwick, M. W., & Schimmel, L. E. (1985). Social Learning intervention to promote metabolic control in type I diabetes mellitus: Pilot experiment results. *Diabetes Care, 8*(2), 152-155.

Kappen, M. J. (1995). *Perceived self-efficacy: A major determinant of diabetes self-management behavior for children with insulin-dependent diabetes mellitus?* Unpublished review paper, Department of Nursing Science, University of Utrecht, The Netherlands.

Kappen, M. J. (1998). *Het ontwikkelen van een meetinstrument dat bij kinderen van 8-12 jaar met insuline-afhankelijke diabetes mellitus self-efficacy beliefs meet ten aanzien van hun diabetes zelfsorg* [Instrument development and testing for self-efficacy beliefs in diabetes management of children 8 to 12 years of age with insulin dependent diabetes mellitus]. Unpublished Master's Thesis, University of Utrecht, The Netherlands.

Kavanagh, D. J., Gooley, S., & Wilson, P. H. (1993). Prediction of adherence and control in diabetes. *Journal of Behavioral Medicine, 16*(5), 509-522.

LaGreca, A. M. (1990). Issues and perspectives on the child assessment process. In A. M. LaGreca (Ed.), *Through the eyes of the child: Obtaining self-reports from children and adolescents* (pp. 3-17). Boston: Allyn and Bacon.

Lynn, M. R. (1986). Determination and quantification of content validity. *Nursing Research, 35*(6), 382-385.

Marshal, S. M., & Barth, J. H. (2000). Standardization of HbA1c measurements: A consensus statement. *Diabetic Medicine, 17,* 5-6.

Maibach, E., & Murphy, D. A. (1995). Self-efficacy in health promotion research and practice: Conceptualization and measurement. *Health Education Research, 10*(1), 37-50.

McCaul, K. D., Glasgow, R. E., & Schafer, L. C. (1987). Diabetes regimen behaviors: Predicting adherence. *Medical Care, 25,* 868-881.

Nunnally, J. C. (1978). *Psychometric theory* (2nd ed.). New York: McGraw-Hill.

Owen, S. (1988). *Short course in instrument development.* Unpublished document, University of Connecticut, Storrs, CT.

Padgett, D., Mumford, E., Hynes, M., & Carter, R. (1988). Meta-analysis of the effects of educational and psychological interventions on management of diabetes mellitus. *Journal of Clinical Epidemiology, 41*(10), 1007-1030.

Pennings-van der Eerden, L. (1992). *Zelfzorggedrag in de behandeling van diabetes mellitus; theorie, meting en determinanten van zelfzorggedrag en diabeteseducatie*

[Self-care behavior in the treatment of diabetes mellitus; theory, measurement and determinants of self-care behavior and diabetes education]. Amsterdam: Thesis Publishers.

Polit, D. F., & Hungler, B. P. (1999). *Nursing research, principles and methods* (6th ed.). Philadelphia: Lippincott.

Reynolds, W. M. (1993). Self-report methodology. In T. H. Ollendick & M. Hersen (Eds.), *Handbook of child and adolescent assessment* (pp. 98-123). Boston: Allyn and Bacon.

Shortridge-Baggett, L. M., & Roden, G. (1994). *Instrument development for management of self-efficacy of diabetes mellitus for newly diagnosed insulin dependent children.* Unpublished document. Lienhard School of Nursing, Pace University, Pleasantville, NY.

Shortridge-Baggett, L. M., & van der Bijl, J. J. (1996). International collaborative research on management self-efficacy in diabetes mellitus. *Journal of the New York State Nurses Association, 27*(3), 9-19.

Sophia Kinderziekenhuis-Sophia Children's Hospital, Diabetes Outpatient Clinic. (1994). De Glyco-Hb of HbA1c test  or [The Glyco-HB or HbA1c test]. *Informatiefolder 2.* Rotterdam, The Netherlands: Sophia Children's Hospital.

Stone, W. L., & Lemanek, K. L. (1990). Developmental issues in children's self-reports. In A. M. LaGreca (Ed.), *Through the eyes of the child: Obtaining self-reports from children and adolescents* (pp. 3-17). Boston: Allyn and Bacon.

Thibodeau, J. A., & Hawkins, J. W. (1988). Developing an original tool for research. *Health Care Issues/Research Focus, 13*(7), 56-59.

# 4

# The Development and Psychometric Testing of an Instrument to Measure Diabetes Management Self-Efficacy in Adolescents With Type 1 Diabetes

Amber Moens
Mieke H. F. Grypdonck
Jaap J. van der Bijl

Diabetes mellitus is a chronic dysfunction of the metabolism of carbohydrates, fat and proteins, which appears as a result of an absolute or relative lack of insulin or as a result of a combination of factors which inhibit the functioning of the insulin. Diabetes is one of the most prevalent chronic illnesses in the western world, affecting 2% to 4% of the population (van Ballegooie, 1995). It is an important health problem in the United States, the Netherlands, and Belgium. In Belgium the incidence of type 1 diabetes mellitus in persons younger than 14 years is 10-14/100,000 a year (Fuller, 1992). In the Netherlands the prevalence of type 1 diabetes mellitus is approximately 1060-1240/100,000 with 100/100,000 for the age group younger than 14 and 200/100,000 for the age group of 14-24 years (CBS, 1998).

The starting point of diabetes treatment for adolescents is active participation of the patient in self-management activities, including glycemic controls and keeping a diary with the results, injecting insulin, adjusting insulin or food doses, and following food prescriptions (Simons, 1992). Those activities are necessary to prevent complications like hypo- and hyperglycemia and damage to the veins in the eyes, kidneys or nervous system.

To teach these activities, many educational programs have been developed. The focus of those programs is on improving skills and attitudes, but this appears to be ineffective in improving glycemic control (Funnell et al., 1991). Self-efficacy has been shown to be an important variable in the self-management of diabetes (Johnson, 1996). Studies of self-efficacy in adolescents with type 1 diabetes have shown a positive relationship between self-efficacy beliefs and metabolic control (Grossman, Brink, & Hauser, 1987), between self-efficacy and adherence (Littlefield et al., 1992; McCaul, Glasgow, & Schafer, 1987; Palardy, Greening, Ott, Holderby, & Atchison, 1998), and between self-efficacy and quality of life (Grey, Boland, Yu, Sullivan-Bolyai, & Tamborlane, 1998). No suitable self-efficacy instrument in

Dutch for adolescents with diabetes mellitus, however, could be located for use in the Netherlands and in Belgium. The study reported here was designed to develop and test a diabetes management self-efficacy instrument for this group.

## METHODS

### Design

The study was conducted in three phases. In the first phase the instrument measuring diabetes management self-efficacy in adolescents with type 1 diabetes was developed. In the second phase the content validity of the instrument was judged. In the third phase the reliability and validity of the instrument were determined.

***Phase 1: Instrument Development.*** Because self-efficacy is task-specific, not personality-specific, a number of items containing diabetes self-management activities relevant to 12- to 18-year-old diabetics had to be formed. The self-management activities which adolescents have to perform daily were derived from the literature and from the diabetes education program of a Belgian hospital (UZ Gasthuisberg). The following self-management activities were selected: injecting insulin, self-control, adjusting to lower and higher sugar levels, arranging meals, and exercising (Saucier & Clarks, 1993).

The concept of self-efficacy consists of three dimensions: level, strength and generality. Maibach and Murphy (1995) have noted that the predictive validity of a self-efficacy instrument is greater when the three dimensions of self-efficacy are included. All three dimensions were integrated in the instrument. On each of the self-management activities mentioned above, a number of items were formulated which on the one hand reflect the specific, often situation-related tasks which adolescents with type 1 diabetes have to perform in order to prevent health complications, and on the other hand express whether patients consider themselves capable to accomplish the task (= the strength dimension of self-efficacy). In English versions of self-efficacy instruments, the expression "How confident are you at . . . " is often used to capture the strength dimension (Maibach & Murphy, 1995). This formulation is hard to use in Dutch. Other phrases are more common in Dutch, such as: "I think I'm able to . . ."; "Do you think you can . . ."; "I'm sure I can. . . ." After consultation with self-efficacy experts, the wording was set as "I'm convinced I can . . ." because this gives a picture of perceived self-efficacy in strong form.

Further, to cover the level dimension of self-efficacy, several difficult diabetes management situations had to be included in the instrument. These difficult situations were identified through focus group interviews with adolescents with type 1 diabetes. Sixteen patients with diabetes between 12 and 18 years old were contacted through physicians and diabetes nurses to take part in the focus groups. None of these participants was hospitalized at that moment. Another four adolescents were contacted to read the instrument and see if there were any difficult questions or words they did not understand. Four focus group interviews were held with four members each. The participants were very open about their self-management behaviors, even when nonadherence was discussed. The following situations seemed to be particularly difficult for the adolescents: not taking candies, adjusting insulin doses or meals in stressful periods (e.g., during exams) or during sports, extra checks of blood glucose when taking a long trip or when sleeping a long time. These difficult situations were integrated into the instrument.

Finally, the generality dimension had to be assured by selecting items representing the different behavorial domains of diabetes self-management. This first phase of instrument development resulted in an instrument containing 30 items about injecting insulin (6 items), nutrition (9 items), regulating diabetes (7 items), hypo- and hyperglycaemia (5 items) and three general items about having diabetes. A 5-point Likert response scale was used:

1. Yes, surely;
2. Probably yes;
3. Maybe yes, maybe no;
4. Probably not;
5. Surely not.

The self-efficacy scores are summed and divided by the total number of items to indicate the strength of perceived self-efficacy for different levels of performance (level or magnitude) regarding the total domain of diabetes self-management activities. Higher scores show less self-efficacy.

***Phase 2: Establishment of Content Validity.*** The content validity of the instrument was established using the method of Lynn (1986). The instrument was sent to 10 experts. Half of the experts had been contacted earlier in the larger project to validate similar instruments for other groups of patients with diabetes; they were all Dutch experts. The other half of the experts were new and were found through the literature and through contacts with Belgian hospitals. The experts were asked to judge the 30 items on a 4-point Likert scale: 4 = very relevant, 3 = relevant but needs a slight change in formulation, 2 = only relevant if the formulation of the item is totally changed, 1 = not relevant at all. The experts were also asked to give comments or suggestions on the items. Finally, they were asked to formulate items that, in their opinion, were missing from the instrument and relevant to diabetes management self-efficacy in adolescents with type 1 diabetes mellitus. An item was accepted as valid if 8 out of 10 experts gave a score of 3 or 4 on the item.

All experts returned their judgments of the instrument. Most experts also made some remarks and/or suggestions to improve the items or gave an explanation for their scores. One expert did not give any score and was, therefore, excluded from the calculation of the content validity. When the Content Validity Index (CVI) of the 30 items was calculated, it was found to be too low ($< .78$) for six items. Two of those items were retained but altered based on comments made on the items. After making these changes and deleting four items, the final instrument had 26 items (see chapter appendix).

*Phase 3: Reliability and Validity Testing—Establishment of Internal Consistency.* To obtain Cronbach's alpha a convenience sample of 130 adolescents with diabetes was contacted to complete the instrument. These adolescents were treated in five different hospitals in Belgium and The Netherlands. Due to the contacts the researcher had with these hospitals, it was relatively easy to get access to this sample. Internal consistency was determined through calculation of Cronbach's alpha. Because self-efficacy may vary across the dimensions, level, strength and generality, however, and in this instrument may vary across different behavioral domains (such as nutrition, exercise, and medical treatment), there was a strong possibility that this instrument contained more than one factor or dimension. In other words, the instrument could be multidimensional instead of homogeneous or unidimensional. Therefore, as recommended by Clark and Watson (1995), mean interitem correlation was used as the criterion for internal consistency; this should be between 0.15 and 0.50.

*Establishment of Construct Validity.* A principal axis factor analysis with oblique rotation was done to determine the possible factors of the instrument. In order to obtain the best fitting structure and the correct number of factors, the following criteria were used: eigenvalues greater than 1.0, factor loadings higher than 0.40 and the so-called scree-plot criterion and elbow criterion regarding the eigenvalues (de Heus, van der Leeden, & Gazendam, 1995).

## RESULTS

### Demographics

Of the 130 instruments sent to adolescents with diabetes, 90 were completed and returned, resulting in a response rate of nearly 70%. Of these 90, six were not usable: four of the respondents were too old or too young and two were not able to answer the questions because of mental disability. Thus 84 instruments were usable for analyses. The respondents were 43% boys and 57% girls. Their mean age was 14.6 years (*SD* = 1.83); 59% of the respondents injected insulin four times a day, 35% injected twice a day and only 6% injected three times a day. The mean duration of illness was 5.8 years (*SD* = 3.27).

### Internal Consistency

Eighty-one instruments were usable for calculating Cronbach's alpha; three instruments had a missing value. Cronbach's alpha for the 26-item instrument was 0.86. Though the alpha value was high, it was not certain that the instrument was homogeneous (De Heus et al.,1995). Therefore, inter-item correlations were calculated. According to Clark and Watson (1995) these should be between 0.15 and 0.50. The mean interitem correlation was 0.34. Only 3 out of 66 interitem correlations fell outside the recommended range of 0.15 to 0.50, indicating the existence of a unidimensional instrument.

## Construct Validity

A principal axis factor analysis without rotation resulted in six factors with eigenvalues greater than one. They accounted for 71% of the variance in scores and referred to the different domains of diabetes management behaviors. With the aid of a scree plot, a more suitable factor extraction was sought. The elbow criterion indicated two twists at factor two and factor four. From the fifth factor onwards the graphical line of the eigenvalues forms more or less a straight line (scree criterion). Therefore, a possible factor solution could vary from two to five factors. Two-, three-, four-, and five-factor extractions were then considered theoretically and empirically. Finally, a two-factor solution was chosen because it appeared to have the best possibilities for interpretation.

The first factor accounted for 24.5% of the variance in scores and the second factor accounted for about 8.8%. In the oblique rotation, the correlation between factors was $r = .34$. The two factors that explained 33.3% of the variance were interpreted as reflecting the two dimensions of the self-efficacy concept: strength and magnitude. Besides estimating how certain he or she is in performing a specific task (strength), the person also judges the difficulty of the task (magnitude). Therefore, patients would be expected to appraise their diabetes management behaviors at at least two levels: general situations and the less general or more difficult self-management situations. The two-factor solution shows this division (see Table 4.1). The first factor includes items reflecting daily diabetes situations regarding medical treatment and nutrition. The second factor consists of items which deal with more difficult situations, like adjusting the insulin dose in the presence of stress, illness or physical exercise. Interestingly, the items with the highest loadings (reflecting less self-efficacy) were identical to aspects of self-management stated as most difficult in the focus group interviews.

Given factor intercorrelations, the Cronbach's alphas of the two factors, and the a priori multidimensional definition of diabetes management self-efficacy, there was some question as to whether the instrument contained two separate subscales. To demonstrate the existence of subscales, intrasubscale item correlations must be systematically higher than the intersubscale item correlations. If this condition cannot be met, then subscales should be abandoned in favor of a single overall score (Clark & Watson, 1995).

The average intercorrelation of the items of Factor 1 (general situations) was .34, whereas that for Factor 2 (difficult situations) was .33. The average correlation of the items between Factor 1 items and Factor 2 items was .34. These findings show that the intrasubscale item correlations were not systematically higher (.34 and .33) than the intersubscale item correlation (.34). Thus there were no substantial data to justify the existence of two subscales.

**TABLE 4.1.** Pattern Matrix of the Factor Loadings for the Two Extracted Factors After Oblique Rotation (*n* = 84)

| | |
|---|---|
| *Factor 1: general diabetes self-management situations* (α = 0.86) | |
| Inject insulin in all situations | 0.72 |
| Follow diet prescriptions all the time OR extra blood sugar check in case of skipping a meal | 0.69 |
| Stick to diet at a party | 0.67 |
| Inject insulin at the right time of the day | 0.66 |
| Take care of diabetes when staying at friends just as well as when being at home | 0.64 |
| Refuse sugared candies when offered by friends | 0.63 |
| Discuss results of good or bad glycemic control with physician | 0.55 |
| Blood sugar control as many times as advised by the diabetic team | 0.53 |
| Regularly consult physician for diabetes control | 0.50 |
| Select the right foods | 0.50 |
| Extra blood sugar control in case of a long trip | 0.48 |
| Eat exactly the right amount of food in case of a hypo | 0.47 |
| | |
| *Factor 2: difficult diabetes self-management situations* (α = 0.72) | |
| Adjust insulin dose when getting up late | 0.67 |
| Adjust insulin dose when having exams | 0.63 |
| Adjust insulin dose in case of illness | 0.50 |
| Adjust insulin dose when going in for sports | 0.46 |
| React correctly in case of forgetting sometimes to inject insulin | 0.46 |

## DISCUSSION AND CONCLUSIONS

The psychometric characteristics of the diabetes management self-efficacy scale for adolescents with type 1 diabetes mellitus are satisfying, and the instrument therefore can be used to assess adolescents' educational needs or evaluate the effectiveness of diabetes education programs. The Cronbach's alpha value of 0.86 indicates that the instrument has an acceptable internal consistency. The interitem correlations give evidence for the unidimensionality of the instrument.

The instrument also has been found content valid. The focus group interviews were especially helpful in revealing the most relevant tasks in diabetes management for adolescents, the complexity of these tasks, and the corresponding challenges.

The factor analysis without rotation showed six factors related to clusters of diabetes self-management activities and reflecting the generality dimension of self-efficacy. The rotated factor solution revealed two factors linked to the strength and magnitude dimensions of self-efficacy. A cautious conclusion, therefore, is that the instrument covers the three dimensions of self-efficacy. A limitation of the factor analysis, however, is the fact that the analysis was done on only 84 patients. The recommendation that at least 10 respondents per item are necessary for factor analysis (Knapp & Campbell, 1989) could not be met, and this may have influenced the findings, in particular the finding of the unidimensionality of the scale.

Future research should focus on analysis of construct and criterion-related validity of the instrument, with data from larger and more diverse samples representing the entire range of the instrument's target population.

## REFERENCES

Ballegooie, E. van. (1995). Maatschappelijke aspecten van diabetes mellitus [Social aspects of diabetes mellitus]. Utrecht: Stichting bio-wetenschappen en maatschappij.

Centraal Bureau voor de Statistiek [CBS]. (1998). *Statistical Yearbook of the Netherlands 1998.* Heerlen/Voorburg: Author.

Clark, L. A., & Watson, D. (1995). Constructing validity: Basic issues in objective scale development. *Psychological Assessment, 7*(3), 309-319.

DeVellis, R. F. (1991). *Scale development theory and applications.* Newbury Park, CA: Sage Publications.

Fuller, J. H. (1992). Recent developments in diabetes epidemiology in Europe. *Health Statistical Quarterly, 45,* 350-354.

Funnell, M., Anderson, R. M., Arnold, M. S., Barr, P. A., Donnelly, M., Johnson, P. D., Taylor-Moon D., &White, N. H. (1991). Empowerment: An idea whose time has come in diabetes education. *The Diabetes Educator,16*(5), 394-400.

Glasgow, R. E., & Osteen, V. L. (1992). Evaluating diabetes education. *Diabetes Care, 15*(10), 1423-1432.

Grey, M., Boland, E. A., Yu, C., Sullivan-Bolyai, S., & Tamborlane, W. V. (1998). Personal and family factors associated with quality of life in adolescents with diabetes. *Diabetes Care, 21*(6), 909-914.

Grossman, H. Y., Brink, S., & Hauser, S. T. (1987). Self-efficacy in adolescent girls and boys with insulin-dependent diabetes mellitus. *Diabetes Care, 10*(3), 324-329.

Heus, P. de, Leeden, R. van der, & Gazendam, B. (1995). *Toegepaste data-analyse: Technieken voor niet-experimenteel onderzoek in de sociale wetenschappen* [Applied data analysis for nonexperimental techniques in the social sciences]. Utrecht: Lemma.

Johnson, S. B. (1984). Knowledge, attitudes, and behavior: Correlates of health in childhood diabetes. *Clinical Psychologie Review, 4,* 503-524.

Knapp T. R., & Campbell-Heider, N. (1989). Numbers of observations and variables in multivariate analyses. *Western Journal of Nursing Research, 11,* 634-641.

Krueger, R. A. (1988). *Focus groups.* Newbury Park, CA: Sage Publications.

Littlefield, H. C., Craves, J. L., Rodin, G. M., Daneman, D., Murray, M. A., & Rydall, A. C. (1992). Relationship of self-efficacy and binging to adherence to diabetes regimen among adolescents. *Diabetes Care, 15*(1), 90-94.

Lynn, M. R. (1986). Determination and quantification of content validity. *Nursing Research, 35,* 382-385.

Maibach, E., & Murphy, D. A. (1995). Self-efficacy in health promotion research and practice: Conceptualization and measurement. *Health Education Research: Theory and Practice, 10*(1), 37-50.

McCaul, K. D., Glasgow, R. E., & Schafer, L. C. (1987). Diabetes regimen behaviors. Predicting adherence. *Medical Care, 25*(9), 868-881.

Palardy, N., Greening, L., Ott, J., Holderby, A., & Atchison, J. (1998). Adolescents' health attitudes and adherence to treatment for insulin-dependent diabetes mellitus. *Journal of Developmental and Behavioral Pediactrics, 19*(1), 31-37.

Polit, D. F., & Hungler, B. P. (1999). *Nursing research: Methods, appraisal and utilization.* Philadelphia: Lippincott.

Saucier, C. P., & Clarks, L. M. (1993). The relationship between self-care and metabolic control in children with insulin-dependent diabetes mellitus. *The Diabetes Educator, 19*(2), 133-135.

Shortridge-Baggett, L., & Bijl, J. J. van der (1996). International collaborative research on management self-efficacy in diabetes mellitus. *Journal of the New York State Nurses Association, 27*(3), 9-14.

Simons, M. R. (1992). Interventions related to compliance. *Nursing Clinics of North America, 27*(2), 477-484.

Stuurgroep Toekomstscenario's Gezondheidszorg. (1990). *Chronische ziekten in het jaar 2005. Deel 1. Scenarios over diabetes mellitus 1990-2005* [Chronic illnesses in the year 2005. Part 1. Scenarios about diabetes mellitus 1990-2005]. Utrecht: Bohn, Scheltema & Holkema.

APPENDIX

# DIABETES MANAGEMENT SELF-EFFICACY SCALE FOR ADOLESCENTS WITH TYPE 1 DIABETES

## Instructions

Hello, as a person with diabetes you have to perform several activities on a day-to-day basis in order to manage your diabetes as well as possible. Some of these activities are performed more successfully than others. The purpose of this scale is to let us know how convinced you are in performing all these activities.

The 26 items of the scale have to do with managing your diabetes. All the items have to be answered by you personally, because we are interested in your opinion about your diabetes management! There are no good or bad answers.

It is of great importance that you read the items carefully and complete all the items.

Every item has five response alternatives. Select the alternative (by marking the response alternative you have selected) which best represents your opinion. Attention, no more than one answer per item is allowed.

*For example*

I'm convinced that I am able to repair a flat tire of my bicycle:

  ( ) yes, surely
  ( ) probably yes
  ( ) maybe yes, maybe no
  (X) probably not
  ( ) no, surely not

If you answer "probably not" (the fourth response alternative), then mark the fourth alternative as shown in the example above.

*Scale Items*

1. I'm convinced that I am able to continually alternate my insulin injection places.
2. I'm convinced that I can inject my insulin in all situations.
3. I'm convinced that I can react correctly in case of forgetting sometimes to inject insulin.
4. I'm convinced that I can inject my insulin at the right time of the day.
5. I'm convinced that I am able to do an extra check of my blood sugar when out for a long time and not able to take my meal directly.
6. I'm convinced that I am able to adjust my insulin dose and/or diet when going in for sports.
7. I'm convinced that I can choose what to eat or not.
8. I'm convinced that I can adjust my insulin dose in relation to my nutritional needs.
9. There are two versions of this question:

Question intended for persons who inject insulin 1 or 2 times a day:

 9a. I'm convinced that I am able to eat all the required meals and snacks.

Question intended for persons who inject insulin 3 or 4 times a day:

9b. I'm convinced that I am able to perform extra blood sugar control in case of skipping a meal or eating at a later point in time.

10. I'm convinced that I can refuse sugared candies when offered by friends.

11. I'm convinced that I am able to keep my diet when going to a party.

12. I'm convinced that I am able to take sufficient exercise regularly or do sports.

13. I'm convinced that I am able to adjust my diet and/or insulin dose correctly when getting up late.

14. I'm convinced that I can carry out regular consults with my physician for diabetes control.

15. I'm convinced that I am able to check my blood sugar as many times as advised by my physician or the diabetes team, and not only when I feel that my blood sugar is too high or too low.

16. I'm convinced that I am able to discuss the results of my blood sugar tests with my physician or with somebody on the diabetes team, even when they are not satisfactory.

17. I'm convinced that I can feel when my blood sugar is too low.

18. I'm convinced that I am able to take Dextro's (or sugar, cookie, coke . . .) with me when I go out.

19. I'm convinced that I can feel when my blood sugar is too high.

20. I'm convinced that I am able to eat a snack in the classroom in case of a hypo, even when my classmates are watching.

21. I'm convinced that I am able to adjust my insulin dose and/or diet when having exams or difficult tests.

22. I'm convinced that I am able to eat exactly sufficient food in case of a hypo.

23. I'm convinced that I dare to tell at a new school that I have diabetes.

24. I'm convinced that I am able to tell my friends what I have to do and not do because of my diabetes.

25. I'm convinced that I can adjust my insulin dose correctly in case of illness.

26. I'm convinced that I am able to manage my diabetes when staying with friends, as well as when I am at home.

# 5

# The Use of Self-Efficacy Enhancing Methods in Diabetes Education in the Netherlands

**Dorine J. E. M. Koopman-van den Berg**
**Jaap J. van der Bijl**

Diabetes mellitus is characterized by abnormalities in glucose metabolism resulting from deficiencies in insulin production, utilization or both, which lead to abnormally high serum glucose levels (van Ballegooie & Heine, 1991). In 1993 the prevalence of diabetes in persons above the age of 30 years was estimated at 2.7% of the Dutch population on the basis of cases reported by general practitioners and at 3.2% based on self-reported cases in surveys. The prevalence increases by 7.1% per life-year for men and by 7.7% for women. The estimated number of people with diabetes in the Netherlands in 1993 ranged between 235,000 and 285,000 (Baan, Bonneux, Ruwaard, & Feskens, 1998), out of a total population of 15 million people. Research done in America (Harris, Hadden, Knowler, & Bennett, 1987) and in the Netherlands (Baan et al., 1998; Grootenhuis, 1994) indicates that only half of all patients with diabetes are registered as such, and systematic screening would increase the prevalence figure 1.5 to 2 times.

The management of diabetes requires an individual to possess a basic knowledge of the disease and the skills necessary to manage the condition. The consequences of poor control include significant microvascular and macrovascular complications, with the potential for life-altering outcomes. The required skills include management of diet, exercise, self-monitoring of blood glucose levels, medication administration, hygiene and avoidance of complications. Traditional diabetic education has been designed to improve knowledge, attitudes and skills and thus to improve compliance with treatment advice. Studies have shown that knowledge alone, however, does not predict individuals' capabilities to incorporate self-management behaviors into their activities of daily living (Glasgow & Osteen, 1992; Nagasawa, Smith, Barnes, & Fincham, 1990). Coping skills are also necessary to manage the day-to-day regimen of diabetes (Rubin, Peyrot, & Saudek, 1993).

## SELF-EFFICACY IN DIABETES EDUCATION

Self-efficacy has been shown to be important in the self-management of diabetes (Johnson, 1996). International studies of self-efficacy enhancing programs used in diabetes education and all national intervention studies in diabetes education were identified through the literature. Three American studies were found and six studies in the Netherlands (van den Berg, 1999). All nine studies gave a description of the target population, although not all in detail. Four programs focused on patients with type 2 diabetes, four on patients with type 1 diabetes, and one program on a group of patients including both types of diabetes. The duration of the programs varied between 4 x 3 hours (de Weerdt, Visser, Kok, & van der Veen, 1989) and a 5-day 37-hour extramural program (Rubin, Peyrot, & Saudek, 1993). Five education programs involved a nurse, and the rest of the programs involved other disciplines.

In all the programs attention was paid to knowledge transfer and skills training, and in five programs the focus was on attitude training, using group discussions and exchanging experiences (van de Arend & Schrijvers, 1996; van Doorn et al., 1994; Engels & Hospers, 1994; van Kemenade et al., 1989; Pennings-van der Eerden, Ripken, van Heijst, & Schrijvers, 1991). All nine programs used mastery experience and two programs included goal setting. Also, three programs reported the use of verbal persuasion in coping-skills training (Glasgow et al., 1992; Grey, Boland, Davidson, Yu, & Tamborlane, 1999; Rubin et al., 1993). This training was designed to help people overcome obstacles to the successful application of new knowledge and skills and to teach people to deal with problems in regimen adherence. In two programs vicarious experience was used (van Kemenade et al., 1989; de Weerdt et al., 1989), in the latter by using video. These two programs also included verbal persuasion by emphasizing people's own responsibility for diabetes management. In two studies self-evaluation was recognizable through attention to stress- and fear-reduction (de Weerdt et al., 1989) and reduction of depression (Rubin et al., 1993).

Nevertheless, in all nine programs self-efficacy-enhancing educational methods could be identified, although the explicit focus of most of these programs was not directed at enhancing self-efficacy. While these studies provide evidence of the use of self-efficacy-enhancing methods in educational programs for persons with diabetes, no study to date has systematically explored the use of these methods. Therefore, the study reported here examined the use of self-efficacy-enhancing educational methods by nurse diabetes educators throughout the Netherlands.

## METHODS

This exploratory study was conducted in two stages. In the first stage a questionnaire was sent to all 445 nurse diabetes educators who were members of the Dutch department of the European Association of Diabetes Educators (EADE), asking what self-efficacy-enhancing educational methods they used in current education programs for people with diabetes mellitus. In the second stage four educational programs were observed, two nurse diabetes educators were interviewed and two course documents were analyzed to examine in more detail how nurse diabetes educators were using the self-efficacy-enhancing educational methods.

The questionnaire sent to all nurse diabetes educators asked eight questions about the nurses (gender, age, education, and occupation) and the courses they deliver (intra-/extramural, individuals/groups, number of courses per year, and so forth), and 15 questions on the use of self-efficacy-enhancing educational methods. These questions were based on the literature about Bandura's four sources of self-efficacy information and information about self-efficacy enhancing strategies used in diabetes education intervention studies (van den Berg, 1999). This resulted in seven questions on the information source, performance accomplishment, two questions on the use of modeling (vicarious experience), four questions regarding the use of verbal persuasion and two questions regarding the information source, self-evaluation (see Table 5.1). The respondents were asked to answer these 15 questions on a 4-point scale (4 = always, 3 = generally, 2 = sometimes, 1 = never). The instrument was sent to three experts, who checked it for readability and validity using the Content Validity Index method (Lynn, 1986). All questions were judged content valid and no alterations were needed.

The results from the questionnaire formed the criteria for selection of nurse diabetes educators and their educational programs to be observed, interviewed or analyzed. The nurses who reported the highest scores on the 15 questions about the use of self-efficacy-enhancing strategies were expected to provide the most useful information about the strategies they used to enhance self-efficacy in their programs, and were asked to participate. Differences in programs (e.g., group or individual education) and target group (e.g., type of diabetes or age group) were also criteria for selection. In total, 5 diabetes nurses were approached to observe their educational programs. One nurse refused to participate because of possible disturbance of the group process due to the observations. Thus, four educational programs were observed: one was an intramural group course, including four sessions of 3 hours; one was an extramural group course, including four sessions of 2 hours; one included a day in an outpatient clinic with individual diabetes education and the fourth was a day of individual extramural education. The observations were made by eight nursing students in the last year of their bachelor's degree programs. A semistructured observation list was used. This list contained the same strategies listed in the questionnaire and was checked by the same three experts. The students received observation training. They independently scored a videotaped diabetes education program. Interobserver reliability was assessed with the help of Fleiss's Kappa. The initial Kappa was 0.50, indicating a reasonable amount of interrater agreement (Bouter & van Dongen, 1991). Differences in observations were discussed and clarified and further assessment of interrater reliability with two observers revealed optimal Kappa scores of 1. To get additional and more detailed information, apart from the observations, two course documents including self-efficacy enhancing methods were also analyzed and two nurse diabetes educators were interviewed. One of them worked only with children.

Descriptive statistics were employed on the data of the questionnaire using SPSS for Windows. The observation lists, course documents and interviews were analyzed using the method of content analysis as described by McCain (1988).

## RESULTS

### Questionnaire

The questionnaire was sent to 445 nurse diabetes educators. The response rate was 59%, thus 261 nurses responded; 94% of the respondents were female and 6% were male. Their average age was 39 years, with a mode of 33 and a standard deviation of 9 years. Ages ranged from 25 to 65 years. Of the respondents, 99% had had additional preparation in the field of diabetes education. Table 5.1 shows the percentages of nurse diabetes educators using the self-efficacy enhancing educational methods listed on the questionnaire. Items within each information category are ordered hierarchically based on the response alternative, "always."

According to self-report all of the 261 respondents regularly made use of self-efficacy-enhancing educational methods. Performance accomplishment strategies were the most used strategies, especially the guided enactment strategies. Goal setting, subdividing complex skills and variety in the complexity of self-management situations were used less. The vicarious experience strategies were the least used strategies in diabetes education. Only 3% of the nurse diabetes educators said that they always or generally used observation of others. Nine percent of the nurse diabetes educators said that they always or frequently used videotapes, if available, in their educational programs. Nearly 80% of the respondents reported additionally that using videos was not possible. The strategies within the information source, verbal persuasion, were also frequently used. Almost all the educators always or generally made use of positive remarks to promote the desired behaviors and they all stressed most of the time the patients' responsibility regarding self-management activities. Coping with difficult situations and involving the partner of the patient in the diabetes education are lesser reported strategies. In the category of self-evaluation, the majority of the nurses provide a calm learning environment. Only 9%, however, reported that they always or generally taught people relaxation techniques or used biofeedback.

### Observations

The questionnaires showed that planning exercises and demonstrating techniques were commonly used methods. This was not confirmed by the observations, however. There was a considerable difference between the results of the questionnaire and the results of the observations. Nurse diabetes educators responding to the questionnaire said they often used the performance accomplishments but this was not confirmed by the observations. Practicing skills and setting goals, for example, were not seen in the educational programs observed.

**TABLE 5.1. Self-Efficacy Enhancing Methods Used by Nurse Diabetes Educators in The Netherlands**

| | Always % | Generally % | Sometimes % | Never % |
|---|---|---|---|---|
| *Performance Accomplishments* | | | | |
| 1. Do you see to it that the exercises lead to the desired outcomes? | 87 | 13 | 0 | 0 |
| 2. During practicing the self-management skills, do you give individual feedback on the patient's actions? | 74 | 23 | 3 | 0 |
| 3. Do you instruct the patient, during the course, to practice certain skills on his own? | 66 | 32 | 2 | 0 |
| 4. Do you point out, during practicing, what aspects of the self-management skill need improvement? | 66 | 25 | 6 | 3 |
| 5. Do you set goals together with the patient regarding the acquired skills? | 18 | 45 | 27 | 10 |
| 6. During acquiring skills do you subdivide complex skills into subskills? | 18 | 45 | 31 | 6 |
| 7. During acquiring skills do you vary the complexity of the situations in which the skills have to be performed? | 14 | 45 | 36 | 5 |
| *Vicarious Experience* | | | | |
| 8. In the case of modeling, do you make use of video tapes demonstrating other patients performing the desired skills? | 4 | 5 | 61 | 30 |
| 9. In the case of acquiring skills, do you make use of other patients demonstrating the desired behavior? | 1 | 2 | 24 | 73 |
| *Verbal Persuasion* | | | | |
| 10. Do you make appreciative or encouraging remarks to the patient to promote the conduct of the expected behavior? | 61 | 37 | 2 | 0 |
| 11. Do you inform the patient that the responsibility for the self-management activities during the diabetes education stays with the patient? | 43 | 50 | 7 | 0 |
| 12. Do you teach patients in your education program to cope with difficult situations regarding diabetes regulation? | 36 | 51 | 12 | 1 |
| 13. Do you involve partners of the patient in your educational program? | 28 | 58 | 14 | 0 |
| *Self-Evaluation of Physiological Responses* | | | | |
| 14. Do you provide a calm learning environment during the education program? | 54 | 43 | 3 | 0 |
| 15. Do you teach the patient relaxation/biofeedback techniques? | 2 | 7 | 44 | 47 |

Modeling was almost never used by the diabetes educators who answered the questionnaire, nor was it observed. Discussion in a class or group session of overall or specific task performances of others were commonly observed. The observations all indicated that verbal persuasion techniques were often used. Both the questionnaires and the observations showed that nurse diabetes educators rarely taught relaxation techniques but they did provide people with a calm learning environment and offer consistent support.

## Interviews

Of the two interviews with nurse educators only one interview revealed additional information about the use of self-efficacy-enhancing strategies compared with the information from the observations. It was the interview with the nurse who provided diabetes education for children with diabetes. Her educational program was organized for children in different age-groups, varying from 0-3 years of age to 17 years and older, including different strategies, for example, family visits with newly diagnosed children and group education with decreasing involvement of the parents when the children get older. Several diabetes self-management activities were practiced, sometimes with the help of games or the computer, but most of the time by learning from each other. Difficult social situations such as going out for dinner, parties and diabetes self-management activities at school were the subject of group discussions,

## Document Analysis

Two course manuals were available for analysis. One manual described the diabetes education activities which were based on the method of interactional learning. This method was based on three didactical principles for group work:

1. Teaching must be based on the group members' own experiences regarding their diabetes activities.
2. Direct emotional involvement of the patients during the learning process, which means that the content of the program must be of direct concern to the participants.
3. Possibility of social comparison. Patients must have the opportunity to share experiences and emotions regarding their diabetes and recognize their impact.

A procedural characteristic of this method is the use of big billboards. On these boards the group members can stick colored cards with questions or statements. The group is then asked to react to these cards and discuss the various questions or statements. In this way active participation of the group members is stimulated and structures the discussion of diverse diabetes topics.

The second manual focused primarily on improvement of knowledge, attitude, social norms and self-efficacy regarding diabetes self-management. It was stated that behavior change could be realized only when a positive attitude and social influence were attained and when self-efficacy was high enough to execute the desired diabetes behavior. No information was given about the strategies to improve self-efficacy, however.

## DISCUSSION

The purpose of this study was to gain an overview of the use of self-efficacy enhancing educational methods by nurse diabetes educators in the Netherlands, including observation and analysis of how diabetes nurses use these methods in their courses. The study gave a fairly good overview of the various self-efficacy-enhancing educational methods that were used, although the questionnaires and the observations were contradictory at some points. For example, unlike the results from the questionnaires, the observations showed that setting goals together with patients was hardly ever done. Setting goals may not be easily done in group courses, but even in individual education, setting goals was not observed. A possible explanation for the differences could be the small number of programs that were observed. Also, giving exercises and setting goals may be done only with newly diagnosed patients, who could have been underrepresented in the settings observed. Finally, the questionnaire could have stimulated socially desirable responses.

Guided enactment and social persuasion were the most used self-efficacy-enhancing strategies. A striking finding was the rare use of modeling. Observing others successfully perform an activity without adverse consequences tends to enhance expectations of mastery. Yet both the questionnaire and observations showed that modeling was almost never used by diabetes educators. Only 3% of the nurse diabetes educators said that they always or generally use observation of others. Clearly, there is much to be gained in the development of diabetes education that makes use of live and symbolic modeling.

According to the Social Cognitive Theory of Bandura (1977), the combination of all four sources of information is most effective in increasing a person's sense of self-efficacy. Bandura states there is some hierarchy in the information sources: performance accomplishment is considered to be the most influential, vicarious experience is considered a little less so and verbal persuasion and self-evaluation influence self-efficacy the least. The analysis of the two program manuals available showed the lack of clear descriptions of the methods used to improve self-efficacy. It is of the highest importance to describe self-efficacy-enhancing methods to nurse diabetes educators in such a way that they can be optimally used.

To date, many evaluations of diabetes education have focused on gaining knowledge and improving metabolic control (van den Berg, 1999). Future research should focus more on patient-teacher interactions and the effectiveness of self-efficacy-enhancing learning methods. In the end this will lead to the development of improved diabetes education programs based on the enhancement of self-efficacy.

## REFERENCES

Arend, I. J. M. van den, & Schrijvers, A. J. P. (1996). Een evaluatie van een educatieprogramma voor type II-diabetespatiënten, dat is ingebed in de zorgverlening [An evaluation of an educational program for patients with type II diabetes, embedded in the health care practice]. *Tijdschrift voor Sociale Gezondheidszorg, 74*(1), 32-38.

Baan, C. A., Bonneux, L., Ruwaard, D., & Feskens, E. J. M. (1998). The prevalence of diabetes mellitus in the Netherlands. *European Journal of Public Health, 8,* 210-216.

Ballegooie, E. van, & Heine, R. J. (1991). *Diabetes Mellitus.* Utrecht: Bunge.

Bandura, A. (1977). Self-efficacy: Toward a unifying theory of behavioral change. *Psychological Review, 84*(2), 191-215.

Berg, D. J. E. M. van den (1999). *Self-efficacy in educatieprogramma's voor diabetespatiënten* [Self-efficacy in educational programs for patients with diabetes]. Nonpublished literature review, Universiteit of Utrecht.

Bouter, L. M., & Dongen, M. C. J. M. van (1991). *Epidemiologisch onderzoek: opzet en interpretatie* [Epidemiological research: Design and interpretation]. Houten/Antwerpen: Bohn, Stafleu, Van Loghum.

Doorn, M. van, Elderen, T. van, & Berting, M. (1994). Effecten van een groepseducatieprogramma voor diabetespatienten [Effects of a group educational program for patients with diabetes]. *Gedrag & Gezondheid, 22*(3), 138-149.

Engels, J. P. G. M., & Hospers, H. J. (1994). Evaluatie van diabeteseducatie in de eerstelijnsgezondheidszorg [Evaluation of diabetes education in the primary health care]. *Tijdschrift voor Sociale Gezondheidszorg, 72,* 253-257.

Funnell, M. M., Anderson, R. M., Arnold, M. S., Barr, P. A., Donnelly, M., Johnson, P. D., Taylor-Moon, D., & White, N. H. (1991). Empowerment: An idea whose time has come in diabetes education. *The Diabetes Educator, 16*(5), 394-400.

Glasgow, R. E., & Osteen, V. L. (1992). Evaluating diabetes education. Are we measuring the most important outcomes? *Diabetes Care, 15*(10), 1423-1432.

Glasgow, R. E., Toobert, D. J., Hampson, S. E., Brown, J. E., Lewinsohn, P. M., & Donnelly, J. (1992). Improving self-care among older patients with type II-diabetes: The "sixty something . . ." study. *Patient Education and Counseling, 19,* 61-74.

Grey, M., Boland, E. A., Davidson, M., Yu, C., & Tamborlane, W. V. (1999). Coping skills training for youths with diabetes on intensive therapy. Applied Nursing Research, 12(1), 3-12.

Grootenhuis, P. A. (1994). *Epidemiological aspects of the Insulin Resistance Syndrome: The Hoorn Study.* Doctoral dissertation, Vrije University, Amsterdam.

Harris, M. I., Hadden, W. C., Knowler, W. C., & Bennet, P. H. (1987). Prevalence of diabetes and impaired glucose tolerance and plasma glucose levels in U.S. population aged 20-74 yrs. *Diabetes, 36*(4), 523-534.

Johnson, J. A. (1996). Self-efficacy theory as a framework for community pharmacy-based diabetes education programs. *The Diabetes Educator, 22,* 237-241.

Kemenade, Y. W. van, Casparie, A. F., & Nievaard, A. C. (1989). De effecten van diabeteseducatie, georganiseerd door de patiëntenvereniging, op attitude en gedrag van de patiënt [The effects of diabetes education, organized by the patient organization, on attitude and behavior of the patient]. *Tijdschrift voor Sociale Gezondheidszorg, 67*(11), 34-35.

Lynn, M. R. (1986). Determination and quantification of content validity. *Nursing Research, 35*(6), 382-385.

McCain, G. C. (1988). Content analysis: A method for studying clinical nursing problems. *Applied Nursing Research, 1*(3), 146-147.

Nagasawa, M., Smith, M. C., Barnes, J. H., & Fincham, F. E. (1990). Meta-analysis of correlates of diabetes patients' compliance with prescribed medication. *Diabetes Educator, 16,* 192-200.

Pennings-van der Eerden, L. J. M., Ripken, T. M. J., Heijst, P. J. M. van, & Schrijvers, A. J. P. (1991). Effecten van een educatieprogramma voor Type II-diabetespatiënten op kennis, zelfzorg, glucoseregulatie en lipidenprofiel [Effects of an educational program for patients with Type II diabetes on knowledge, self-care, glucose regulation and lipids profile]. *Gedrag & Gezondheid, 19*(5), 246-260.

Rubin, R. R., Peyrot, M., & Saudek, C. D. (1993). The effects of a diabetes education program incorporating coping skills training on emotional well-being and diabetes self-efficacy. *The Diabetes Educator, 19*(3), 210-214.

Weerdt, I. de, Visser, A. P., Kok, G., & Veen, E. A. van der. (1989). Randomized controlled evaluation of an education program for insulin-treated patients with diabetes: Effects on psychosocial variables. *Patient Education and Counseling, 14*(3), 191-215.

# 6

# Strategies Enhancing Self-Efficacy in Diabetes Education: A Review

## Katja E. W. van de Laar
## Jaap J. van der Bijl

The regimen for persons with a chronic illness such as diabetes is complex and lifelong and it demands many changes in behavior, making compliance difficult. Further, the advantages of the diabetes regimen can be seen only in the long term; in the short term the regimen simply causes discomfort. Traditional diabetes education, which focuses on the transfer of information, often does not result in the desired changes in behavior (van Doorn, 1993; Glasgow & Osteen, 1992). Indeed, most educational programs show improvements in knowledge but have little effect on behavior. Also, they rarely lead to improvements in the patient's metabolic parameters (Brown, 1988, 1990, 1992; van Doorn, van Elderen, & Berting, 1994).

The theory of self-efficacy, developed by Bandura as a part of social learning theory, offers a basis for improving the effectiveness of diabetes education because of its focus on changing behavior. Indeed, according to Bandura (1986), self-efficacy is the most important predictor of change in behavior. Padgett, Mumford, Hynes, and Carter (1988), who did a meta-analysis of published and unpublished literature on educational and psychosocial interventions with persons with diabetes, concluded that studies making use of social learning theory had the best results. Similarly, Hurley and Shea (1992) and Hockmeyer (1990) found that persons with high self-efficacy were better able to manage their diabetes self-care, and Hockmeyer's study showed that self-efficacy predicted 64% of the diabetes self-care behaviors. Also Visser, Spijker, Smelt, and Van der Kar (1994) noted that the level of self-care of persons with diabetes depends on their estimation of their self-efficacy. Clearly self-efficacy is important in managing diabetes, and it can be used to predict the self-care behaviors of persons with diabetes (Johnson, 1996; Maddux, Brawley, & Boykin, 1995; Rosenstock, 1985). Enhancing self-efficacy is thus important in diabetes education. Rosenstock (1985) and Johnson (1996) suggest that enhancing self-efficacy should be part of the design of all educational programs for persons with diabetes.

Enhancement of a person's self-efficacy is based on four sources of information: performance accomplishments, vicarious learning, verbal persuasion, and self-appraisal of emotional and physiological responses (Bandura 1977, 1986,

1997). In forming a judgment of efficacy, persons have to weigh and integrate information from the different sources (Bandura, 1986). Strategies to enhance self-efficacy have been described in the literature for each of these four sources of self-efficacy information. This review provides an overview of specific strategies that can be used in these four areas.

## SELF-EFFICACY ENHANCING STRATEGIES

### Performance Accomplishments

Self-efficacy can be enhanced by practicing the intended behavior or task. Experiences of success are the most effective way to develop a strong sense of self-efficacy. They provide evidence that a person can succeed and show the exertions that success costs. Negative experiences disrupt the feeling of self-efficacy, especially when a failure takes place before a stabile sense of self-efficacy has been developed (Bandura, 1995).

Often a task is very complicated, which makes it useful to split up the task or intended behavior into parts which are easy to master. Specific behaviors should then be put in a sequence in order to master each part in turn, first the easy tasks, then the more difficult tasks, until the eventual aim has been reached: the total task. In order to attain this, the intended behavior should be studied carefully to identify the specific aspects of the task which require development of skills (Bandura, 1997; Strecher, DeVellis, Becker, & Rosenstock, 1986). Then start with a task at which the patient certainly can succeed. As noted above, people need experiences of success to improve their self-efficacy (Gonzalez, Goeppinger, & Lorig, 1990). Rapid successes are beneficial to self-efficacy. Failure in an early stage is disadvantageous. Repeating a single task until the patient has mastered it eventually leads to success.

When training persons with diabetes to inject themselves with insulin, the injection process can be split up into much smaller steps. Then each step can be learned by means of repetition. This allows patients to build self-efficacy at each step. After this, the steps can be put together and self-efficacy built for the total process (Baranowski, Perry, & Parcel, 1997). Also, the process of learning self-regulation can be divided into smaller steps. This allows new fields to be explored and practiced (van Doorn, 1993). Johnson (1996) says that persons with diabetes should be allowed time and opportunity to try out a blood-glucose monitoring device until they are successful. Furthermore, they should practice first in simple situations, and later in more complex situations (Bandura, 1986). This means first injecting themselves at home under supervision, and extending this until they can inject themselves in all kinds of different situations.

An important basis for self-efficacy is the person's attribution of previous successes or failures. A person who attributes success to a stable cause—for instance, capacities—has a higher expectation of success in a similar new task, while a person who attributes success to an unstable cause such as luck will not have a higher expectation of success. Similarly, a person who attributes failure to a stable cause will have a lower expectation of success for similar tasks. Attribution of failure to an unstable cause will not decrease the expectation of success. Thus self-efficacy can be enhanced by attributing failure to unstable causes and attributing success to stable causes (Kok et al., 1990).

Persons with diabetes need to be told that positive results, like improvements in blood glucose, are caused by their own exertions, and not by accident or by professional help (van Doorn, 1993). According to Bandura (1986) self-efficacy influences the attributions people make about the causes of their success. Once people have built up high self-efficacy, they are inclined to attribute their success to stable factors and their failures to unstable factors. This again is useful for maintaining high self-efficacy.

Sometimes people interpret their successes negatively. They do not see them, do not want to know about them, or underestimate their importance. In these cases, it is important to help patients experience a success, interpret it as a success, and regard it as their own achievement (Maddux et al., 1995). The importance of establishing goals to enhance self-efficacy is clear. Goal-setting directs and causes motivation for a desired behavior (Bandura, 1986). A negative discrepancy between current achievement level and the desired standard can activate people. Goals influence achievement because they motivate people to exert themselves again and thus they persevere longer in their task. Goals also direct patients' attention, enhance their concentration and lead to new strategies for succeeding. Goals should be specific and sufficiently challenging, rather than easy. Goals also have to be realistic and achievable. Short-term goals are more motivating than long-term ones (Locke, Saari, Shaw, & Latham, 1981).

Self-efficacy can be enhanced by having patients set goals for specific behaviors in the form of a contract with themselves. The client, not the professional, has to decide which kind of behavior needs to be attained. This serves to motivate the client to try to reach the goals. A goal should be clear and specific, and should describe the desired behavior, including the number of attempts which may be necessary to fulfill the task. This specificity helps to make the goal realistic and achievable (Bandura, 1986; Gonzalez, Goeppinger, & Lorig, 1990; Locke et al., 1981).

It is also useful to set concrete goals together with the patient and to set a time for the patient to acquire experience (van Doorn, 1993). After each education session, the contract should be discussed and new goals set by the client (Gonzalez et al., 1990). To enhance their chances for success, patients should be able to get feedback on their achievements and make intermediate corrections on their contract (Gonzalez et al., 1990). Bandura and Cervone (1983) note the importance of feedback on achievements. The combination of setting goals in a contract and giving feedback enhances self-efficacy. Before every education session, feedback should be given on the goals of the preceding period, and clients should report their achievements. At least 30% of each education session should be used for contracts and feedback. Regular contact by phone to ask about the patient's achievements can also be effective (Gonzalez et al., 1990).

A diabetes diary is a good source of feedback for persons with diabetes. Blood-glucose values, the self-care actions and the surrounding circumstances can be noted in the diary, and the patient can thus gain insight into self-regulation (van Doorn, 1993). The diary can also serve as an aid in education (Johnson, 1996). By looking at variations in daily circumstances and the changes in the blood-glucose level that accompany these variations, the patient can see which factors influence blood-glucose, including psychosocial circumstances.

Enhancing the patient's self-efficacy is important. When clients know what is expected of them, are conscious of what will happen to them, and are able to choose behavior strategies, their self-efficacy is enhanced. Clients are then less dependent and more inclined to make internal attributions for their successes (Maddux et al., 1995).

## Vicarious Learning

The second way of developing self-efficacy is vicarious learning, that is, observing other persons' experiences. The person's own capacities are then judged in relation to that other person's achievements. Some people are particularly sensitive to this way of developing self-efficacy, especially people who are insecure or have little experience (Bandura, 1997). Seeing comparable others persevere and succeed in a difficult task strengthens these patients' idea that they can do it themselves. Conversely, seeing others fail in spite of hard efforts, can strengthen patients' doubts about their own capacities. The force of this source of information about self-efficacy is strongly influenced by comparability of the models (Bandura, 1995).

Comparability of models is based on two criteria: shared experiences and similar personal characteristics. Persons with a comparable lifestyle, like friends or colleagues, can serve as models, and models can show skills for the intended behavior. Models who succeed slowly, by trial and error, are better than those who succeed instantly, without problems (Schunk & Carbonari, 1984). Some models can be counterproductive; for instance, models with many more capacities can be seen as out of reach. The best model is a person who has problems, who fights to surmount them and who adapts from day to day. This is a person with whom most people can identify (Gonzalez et al., 1990).

Similar characteristics also have a positive influence, although these character-istics may have nothing to do with the behavior at issue. Comparability in sex, age, ethnic background, socio-economic status or educational level usually are seen as indicators of a person's own capacities (Schunk & Carbonari, 1984). The differ-ences between persons with diabetes are large. Age can vary widely, but other characteristics can also be very different. Role models should be chosen in accordance with this. The suitable models are persons who have diabetes themselves. In group education, selection of patients who have mutual characteristics enables group members to identify with each other (van Doorn, 1993). One possibility is to choose persons with the same health problems, like diabetes. For each problem the group leader can ask the group members for solutions or ideas, and thus group members can be encouraged to help each other in solving their problems. The group members then have the experience that they are experts and they are not always dependent on professionals. Also, they may offer innovative solutions that have not been thought of by professionals (Gonzalez et al., 1990). Modeling can also be used with other educational media like television, videos, brochures and textbooks. Use of models who are comparable to the patient in experiences and characteristics is important (Gonzalez et al., 1990; Schunk & Carbonari, 1984). Bandura (1997) mentions symbolic modeling and emphasizes the effects of television and other visual media on self-efficacy.

A number of investigations have looked at movies as a strategy for vicarious learning. In these films, comparable others carried out specific operations or behaviors in the correct manner. Control groups were shown a movie which had nothing to do with these actions or behaviors. The movies which made use of modeling produced more of the desired change in behavior (Gilbert et al., 1982; Melamed & Siegel, 1975). Several investigations have also tested the use of video tapes to enhance self-efficacy. On the videos the desired behavior was demonstrated using comparable models whenever possible. The investigations all found an increase in self-efficacy (Gist, Schwoerer, & Rosen, 1989; Gortner & Jenkins, 1990; Gross, Fogg, & Tucker, 1995).

According to Johnson (1996), videos can show all aspects of diabetes care and specific role models can be used for different demographic groups, like children, teenagers and older persons with diabetes. A special kind of modeling that can enhance self-efficacy is "self-modeling." This technique helps patients change their behavior after seeing a video of themselves showing the desired behavior. The rationale for this approach is that people are interested in videos of themselves which makes them pay attention to the video. Also, people intend to imitate behavior that is adaptive. Seeing faults and negative feedback on a video can be damaging. Self-modeling is a form of "feed-forward," showing people how things should be done. Self-modeling has been used in learning many kinds of skills, including physical skills and communication skills (Dowrick, 1983). For persons with diabetes, self-modeling could be used to learn practical skills and to deal with anxiety.

Role playing is used most often in group education. In role playing the desired behavior is demonstrated and observed. Participants also have an opportunity to practice a behavior and to get feedback from group members and group leaders (Grey et al., 1998; Kaplan, Chadwick, & Schimmel, 1985; Ozer & Bandura, 1990). Grey and colleagues and Kaplan and associates used video recordings of role play by teenagers with type 1 diabetes, since this group is very sensitive to such an approach. Difficult situations and possible solutions were acted out in role plays, recorded on video and afterwards discussed in the group. In this way optimal identification with contemporaries was encouraged and self-efficacy, enhanced. Brown and colleagues (1997) used an interactive video game to enhance self-care among children with diabetes. The children took the roles of animal characters who managed their diabetes themselves, measuring blood glucose, injecting insulin and choosing food. This investigation showed an increase in self-efficacy.

A final form of learning by observation is demonstrations of specific skills or behavior. Nurses, educators or course leaders can demonstrate specific actions. Part of the self-efficacy enhancing protocol used to prepare persons for an operation is demonstration of the desired behaviors by nurses (Oetker-Black, Teeters, Cukr, & Rininger, 1997). Skills like injecting insulin and measuring blood glucose can also be demonstrated (Johnson, 1996).

## Verbal Persuasion

Verbal persuasion is the most commonly used source of information for enhancing self-efficacy. Patients are told that they have the capacity to succeed, since persons will have more confidence in themselves if others have confidence in their capacities. This conviction can cause patients to make more efforts and persevere in a task until the desired behavior has been mastered. Self-strengthening sugges-tions enhance the development of skills and eventually, self-efficacy (Bandura, 1995). This source has limited power in itself, but it is often used in combination with other sources (Bandura, 1997).

Verbal persuasion may also stimulate persons to set higher goals than they would have done by themselves. These goals should remain realistic and attain-able. If goals are not realistic, patients get discouraged by disappointing results (Gonzalez et al., 1990). Positive feedback can also be seen as a kind of persuasion (Gonzalez et al., 1990). Positive feedback is an important reward to induce patients to show a specific behavior and keep it up (den Boer, 1993). It is important, of course, to attribute success to the patient's own efforts.

The success of persuasive communication in changing insights is strongly influenced by the estimated reliability of the source. The more reliable the person who is communicating the message, the greater the success in changing attitudes or learning a new behavior. Estimation of reliability is influenced by three factors: expertise, credibility and attractiveness. Patients experience more feelings of efficacy if they are convinced by a reliable person than if the person is someone they do not trust. Also, people are more easily influenced by a person with knowledge on the topic. Finally the characteristics of the educator, including attractiveness and friendliness, are important (Baron, Byrne, & Kantowitz, 1981). Bandura (1997) mentions the importance of credibility and expertise of the educator. Confidence can also arise from observed equality with the educator; for instance, shared experiences or mutual characteristics enable persons to identify with the educator (Schunk & Carbonari, 1984). Patients can also stimulate each other. This fact can be used in group education. Patients who are experiencing difficulties in a specific area often can be influenced by a group (Gonzalez et al., 1990).

Verbal persuasion to enhance self-efficacy has been tested in several investigations, mostly in the form of positive feedback (Gross et al., 1995; Ozer & Bandura, 1990; Taal, 1995). Oetker-Black and colleagues (1997) used a self-efficacy enhancing protocol to achieve a desired behavior before and after an operation. The nurse gave cognitive instructions for the desired behavior and the motives behind it and tried to convince the patients of the necessity of the behavior. No significant improvements in self-efficacy were found, however. Gortner and Jenkins (1990) used verbal persuasion to enhance self-efficacy through weekly telephone calls to patients who were recovering at home from a heart operation and had to perform physical activities for their recovery. Verbal persuasion techniques were used to influence people to have more confidence in themselves. Self-efficacy was found to be a significant predictor of self-reported activity.

For persons with diabetes, verbal persuasion primarily consists of the transfer of knowledge: patients need to know what is the matter before they can be convinced to change their behavior. Once patients have insight into the reasons why they have to change their behavior and know how they have to change, they need to be stimulated to start making changes in their behavior. For persons with diabetes the changes include changes in diet, weight loss, physical exercise, learning to inject insulin, and learning to measure blood glucose and to interpret the measurements. Instructions can be given on blood-glucose monitoring and on the use of the blood-glucose monitoring device; explanations can also be given on the recommended frequency of monitoring. Patients then have to be observed and encouraged in this behavior (Johnson, 1996). Positive feedback on the actions they have taken and a positive interpretation of possible faults can enhance self-efficacy. Also, people can be encouraged to set their goals higher—for instance, toward more physical exercise or a stricter diet.

## Self-Appraisal of Emotional and Physiological Responses

The fourth source of self-efficacy is the information people obtain from self-appraisal of their physiological and emotional situation. Persons who feel stressed will judge their self-efficacy more negatively than persons who feel relaxed. Also, a positive mood increases self-efficacy and a negative mood decreases it. Self-efficacy can be increased by improving the patient's physical situation, reducing stress, and decreasing negative emotions, as well as by correcting false interpretations of the patient's physical situation. The intensity of emotional and physical reactions is not as important as the way in which they are observed and interpreted. When persons have high self-efficacy, they see a certain tension as a stimulant to achieve, but persons who have doubts experience tension as a restraint.

Maddux and colleagues (1995) claim that persons have more confidence in their own abilities when they feel relaxed. Strategies that reduce and control emotional tension can thus enhance self-efficacy, especially when learning new behavior. The strategies used most often are hypnosis, biofeedback, relaxation training, meditation and medication. One investigation studied the influence of relaxation exercises on self-efficacy with persons who were afraid of a gastroendoscopy. Audio tapes were played to patients informing them that this was a relaxation exercise which would decrease their tension before a gastroendoscopy. The relaxation exercise consisted of intense muscle relaxation and meditation (Gattuso, Litt, & Fitzgerald, 1992). The training showed a positive effect, especially when the relaxation was combined with positive feedback.

Physical symptoms can be seen as indicators of personal ineffectiveness, and changing these interpretations is important. Health care professionals need to determine what people believe and why they believe it, and, if possible, help people change their beliefs. When a specific belief has been identified, the health care professional can start to reinterpret. Double messages should be avoided, and language should be simple and clear. New insights can give patients a new view of their illness. They can also influence a person's judgment of his or her ability to deal with illness (Gonzalez et al., 1990).

Persons with diabetes have to learn to anticipate disturbances of blood glucose by stress, food, and physical exercise. Stress can influence diabetes regulation and lead to metabolic disorders. Physiological stressors like pain and trauma produce heightened insulin intolerance, and so do psychological stressors like undesired life events and daily worries. Suffering with diabetes mellitus automatically leads to some stress. Patients must be medically treated for the rest of their lives, they are subject to numerous threats, and they are daily confronted with their illness. Not surprisingly, persons with diabetes often have a relatively strong sense of fear. How they react to this depends on their knowledge of the illness and their education, as well as motivation, personality and social support.

Three types of fear often occur: fear to inject, fear of complications and fear of hypoglycemia. Health care professionals need to be aware of these fears. Excessive fear is physically taxing for patients and can prevent optimal blood glucose regulation. To decrease the effects of fear, a number of relaxation exercises have been tried with persons with diabetes. Several investigations have shown a positive effect of biofeedback and fear management training, but the investigations had many limitations. Special awareness training programs have also been developed for dealing with the fear of hypoglycemia. Recognition of the fear is important and support should aim at enhancing the patient's sense of control and self-confidence (Ballegooie & Heine, 1995). Johnson (1996) indicates that having patients feel relaxed is also important. Education thus should be given in a relaxed and stress-free environment, because fear and distress have a negative effect on self-efficacy.

Clearly, physiological indicators of self-efficacy play a large part in health functioning. This source of self-efficacy, however, should be seen in the context of the other three sources, which are more concrete and can be better measured.

## Combination of Sources

In forming a judgment of self-efficacy the information from the four sources has to be integrated. The influence of the different sources, however, can differ in each situation and for each person, and few investigations have looked at multidimensional efficacy information (Bandura, 1997).

Maddux and Lewis (1995) claim that combining different sources of self-efficacy is best for enhancement of self-efficacy, and combining all four sources is most effective. Also, Bandura (1986, 1997) mentions that a combination of sources produces the best results, and the combination of practicing and observing others is especially useful. When observing others, patients can study the new skill and gain confidence that they can do it themselves. When this is practiced under supervision, the best effects for self-efficacy are achieved (Schunk & Carbonari, 1984).

A self-efficacy enhancing protocol aimed at preparing patients for an operation and postoperative recovery used a combination of the first three sources of self-efficacy. The nurse gave instructions about the desired behavior and demonstrated the behavior. The patients were asked to also demonstrate the expected behavior until they knew how to do it. Also, the educators tried to verbally convince patients that they were capable of performing the behavior; this did not, however, result in significant improvements in self-efficacy (Oetker-Black et al., 1997).

Ozer and Bandura (1990) developed a program to enhance self-efficacy for women to defend themselves against sexual violence using the first three sources of self-efficacy information. The women were taught special defense techniques, first by demonstrating the necessary techniques, which the women then practiced in simulated situations. The participants all observed each others' exercises so they could learn from each other. After each exercise feedback was given both by the instructors and by participants. One result of the program was an increase in self-efficacy.

Another program tried to enhance the self-efficacy of parents of children with behavioral problems, again using the first three sources of self-efficacy information. Parents watched a number of videotapes in which models were parents with their children in typical family situations. The videotape was stopped at a few specific moments and the parents were asked to discuss the problems and propose solutions. Every week the participants had take-home assignments in which they had to apply the solutions. In addition both the group members and the group leaders made use of verbal persuasion. This program resulted in a significant increase in parental self-efficacy (Gross et al., 1995). A follow-up investigation after 1 year showed that the increase in self-efficacy had been maintained (Tucker, Gross, Fogg, Delaney, & Lapporte, 1998).

A health education program to enhance self-care in patients with cystic fibrosis also used social learning theory. This program focused on observation of others and verbal persuasion, combined with practicing. The patients had to draw up targets themselves, keep a diary and get feedback on their progress. When creating models for observation the characteristics of the client groups were taken into account (Bartholomew et al., 1991). Finally, Taal (1995), in developing an educational program for patients with rheumatoid arthritis, found that the most effective combination was practicing, observing others, and verbal persuasion. For the exercises targets are set, which are laid down in a contract. The program had a favorable effect on self-efficacy, even in a follow-up investigation after 14 months.

Johnson (1996) recommends using self-efficacy theory in developing educational programs for persons with diabetes. All four sources of self-efficacy information should be used with different learning methods. For example, when people are learning to measure and interpret blood glucose, the educator first has to explain the advantages of these measurement and supply the necessary knowledge. The equipment and procedure then can be demonstrated, after which the persons with diabetes have an opportunity to practice at home. This procedure should be repeated until the persons with diabetes are successful. Convincing patients of their capacities is important. Also, Johnson mentions the importance of a relaxed and stress-free environment, because fear can have a negative effect on self-efficacy. Videotapes of all aspects of diabetes care can be shown and special role models can be used for different demographic groups.

Wing, Epstein, Nowalk, Koeske, and Hagg (1985) investigated the effects of a behavioral program on weight loss for patients with type 2 diabetes, using elements of the first three sources of self-efficacy information. The patients got information on nutrition and physical exercise and learned a number of strategies for changing their behavior. Participants had to set targets themselves and keep a diary. Meetings were used to practice and discuss progress, and participants were given assignments to carry out at home. Role-play allowed observation of others. The result was a significant loss of weight during the first 4 months, but this was poorly sustained. After 16 months the effects of the program had disappeared.

Padgett (1991), who investigated factors related to self-efficacy, concluded that persons with higher self-efficacy share a number of characteristics. Younger persons, males, and higher educated persons usually have higher self-efficacy than older persons, women and persons with less education. Persons inclined to depression tend to have lower self-efficacy. Clearly, identifying individual risk factors can increase the effectiveness of interventions to enhance self-efficacy.

Grey and coinvestigators (1998) found that training in coping skills had a positive effect on self-efficacy among teenagers with diabetes. The training was aimed at avoiding inappropriate coping and establishing more positive coping and behaviors. Participants were trained based on the elements of social learning theory, using modeling, verbal persuasion and practice of skills.

When people change behavior, maintenance of the desired behavior is critical. Relapse prevention theory includes high-risk situations in which a person is inclined to relapse to an old habit. To deal with such situations the person needs a coping response, that is, a good way to deal with the situation, preferably devised in advance. Absence of a coping response will lead to lower self-efficacy and relapse. Correct use of a coping response will lead to success, which enhances self-efficacy (Marlatt & Gordon, 1985).

Attributions of success and failure play a part in this respect. Attributions of failure to stable factors like skills and willpower will lead to lower self-efficacy and relapse. In the learning process relapse often occurs. Most people learn by trial and error. A good attribution of the temporary relapse can lead to the desired behavior. Success experiences lead to higher self-efficacy for the specific activity. Thus good coping responses and good attributions can enhance self-efficacy, and they can be learned through the four sources of self-efficacy (Bandura, 1997; Kok et al., 1990).

## CONCLUSIONS

Persons with diabetes can do much of their treatment themselves; usually changes in behavior are necessary, however. Interventions based on Bandura's social cognitive theory show the best results. The concept of self-efficacy appears to be especially important in changing behavior. Several investigations have shown that patients with high self-efficacy show more compliance with regard to their life rules regarding self-management than patients with low self-efficacy. Enhancing self-efficacy is thus a part of diabetes education. Self-efficacy can be enhanced through four sources of self-efficacy information: practicing, observations of others, verbal persuasion and physiological information. For each source, numerous interventions have been described in the literature. Few investigations, however, have studied the effects of the separate sources or looked at the most appropriate combination of sources. Self-efficacy-enhancing programs have not made it clear why they chose the sources or interventions they did. Also, they usually have not elaborated on the way interventions were carried out. Persons with diabetes need to make many behavior changes with regard to self-care. These changes can cause a lot of stress and insecurity, and enhancing self-efficacy can be important. Self-efficacy, however, is not a general feeling but is specific to a task and context. For each aspect of diabetes self-care, self-efficacy has to be built up. Each skill the patient has to master should be specified clearly. An educational program that is designed for all persons with diabetes is not feasible because the diabetes population is so varied, in age, form of diabetes, treatment of diabetes, demographic data, and so forth. Also, the starting level of self-efficacy differs for each task and for each patient. Interventions that make use of combinations of sources, and especially a combination of the first three sources, appear to be most effective. The fourth source, physiological information, is less concrete but can play an important part in enhancing self-efficacy. Educational programs designed to enhance self-efficacy should also be attuned to the patient's individual needs.

# REFERENCES

Ballegooie, E. van, & Heine, R. J. (1995). *Diabetes mellitus.* Utrecht: Bunge.

Bandura, A. (1977). Self-efficacy: A unifying theory of behavioral change. *Psychological Review, 84*(2), 191-215.

Bandura, A. (1986). *Social foundations of thought and action: A social cognitive theory.* Englewood Cliffs, NJ: Prentice Hall.

Bandura, A. (1995). *Self-efficacy in changing societies.* Cambridge: Cambridge University Press.

Bandura, A. (1997). *Self-efficacy, the exercise of control.* New York: W. H. Freeman and company.

Bandura, A., & Cervone, D. (1983). Self-evaluative and self-efficacy mechanisms governing the motivational effects of goal systems. *Journal of Personality and Social Psychology, 45*(5), 1017-1028.

Baranowski, T., Perry, C. L., & Parcel, G. S. (1997). How individuals, environments, and health behavior interact: Social learning theory. In K. Glanz, F. M. Lewis, & B. K. Rimer (Eds.), *Health behavior and health education: Theory, research and practice* (2nd ed., pp. 161-183). San Francisco: Jossey-Bass Publishers.

Baron, R. A., Byrne, D., & Kantowitz, B. H. (1981). *Psychology: Understanding behavior.* Tokyo: Holt-Saunders International Editions.

Bartholomew, L. K., Parcel, G. S., Seilheimer, D. K., Czyzewski, D., Spinelli, S. H., & Congdon, B. (1991). Development of a health education program to promote the self-management of cystic fibrosis. *Health Education Quarterly, 18*(4), 429-443.

Boer, D. J. den (1993). Gedragsbehoud [Behavior preservation]. In V. Damoiseaux, H. T. van der Molen & G. J. Kok (Eds.), *Gezondheidsvoorlichting en gedragsverandering* [Health education and behavior change] (pp. 308-318). Assen, the Netherlands: Van Gorcum.

Brown, S. A. (1988). Effects of educational interventions in diabetes care: A meta-analysis of findings. *Nursing Research, 37*(4), 223-230.

Brown, S. A. (1990). Studies of educational interventions and outcomes in diabetic adults: A meta-analysis revisited. *Patient Education and Counseling, 16,* 189-215.

Brown, S. A. (1992). Meta-analysis of diabetes patient education research: Variations in intervention effects across studies. *Research in Nursing and Health, 15,* 409-419.

Brown, S. J., Lieberman, D. A., Gemeny, B. A., Fan, Y. C., Wilson, D. M., & Pasta, D. J. (1997). Educational videogame for juvenile diabetes: Results of a controlled trial. *Medical Informatics, 22*(1), 77-89.

Doorn, M. van, Elderen, T. van, & Berting, M. (1994). Effecten van een groepseducatie-programma voor diabetespatiënten [Effects of a group educational program for patients with diabetes]. *Gedrag en Gezondheid, 22*(3), 138-149.

Doorn, M. van (1993, August). Bevordering van self-efficacy is een belangrijke stap naar zelfregulatie van diabetes [Enhancement of self-efficacy is a major step in the self-regulation of diabetes]. *Euorpean Association of Diabetes Educators Nieuwsbrief, 8*(3), 25-29.

Dowrick, P. W. (1983). *Using Video.* New York: John Wiley & Sons Ltd.

Gattuso, S. M. Litt, M. D., & Fitzgerald, T. E. (1992). Coping with gastrointestinal endoscopy: Self-efficacy enhancement and coping style. *Journal of Consulting and Clinical Psychology, 1,* 133-139.

Gilbert, B. O., Bennett-Johnson, S., Spiller, R., McCallum, M., Silverstein, J. H., & Rosenbloom, A. (1982). The effect of a peer-modeling film on children learning to self-inject insulin. *Behavior Therapy, 13,* 186-193.

Gist, M. E., Schwoerer, C., & Rosen, B. (1989). Effects on alternative training methods on

Self-efficacy and performance in computer software training. *Journal of Applied Psychology, 74,* 884-891.

Glasgow, R. E., & Osteen, V. L. (1992). Evaluating diabetes education. Are we measuring the most important outcomes? *Diabetes Care, 15*(10), 1423-1432.

Gonzalez, V. M., Goeppinger, J., & Lorig, K. (1990). Four psychosocial theories and their application to patient education and clinical practice. *Arthritis Care, 3,* 132-143.

Gortner S. R., & Jenkins, L. S. (1990). Self-efficacy and activity level following cardiac surgery. *Journal of Advanced Nursing, 15,* 1132-1138.

Grey, M., Boland, E. A., Davidson, M., Yu, C., Sullivan-Bolyai, S., & Tamborlane, W. V. (1998). Short-terms effects of coping skills training as adjunct to intensive therapy in adolescents, *Diabetes Care, 21*(6), 902-908.

Gross, D., Fogg, L., & Tucker, S. (1995). The efficacy of parent training for promoting positive parent-toddler relationships. *Research in Nursing & Health, 18,* 489-499.

Hockmeyer, M. T. (1990). *The influence of self-efficacy and health beliefs, considering treatment mode, on self-care behavior of adults diagnosed within 3 years with non-insulin-dependant diabetes mellitus.* Unpublished doctoral dissertation, University of Maryland.

Hurley, A. C., & Shea, C. A. (1992). Self-efficacy: Strategy for enhancing diabetes self-care. *The Diabetes Educator, 18*(2), 146-150.

Johnson, J. A.(1996). Self-efficacy theory as a framework for community pharmacy-based diabetes education programs. *The Diabetes Educator, 22*(3), 237-241.

Kaplan, R. M., Chadwick, M. W., & Schimmel, L. E. (1985). Social learning intervention to promote metabolic control in type I diabetes mellitus: Pilot experiment results. *Diabetes Care, 8*(2), 152-155.

Kok, G. J., Vries, H. de, Boer, D.J. de, Dijkstra, M., Gerards, F., Hospers, H. J., & Mudde, A. (1990). De rol van eigen effectiviteit bij de beïnvloeding van gezondheidsgedrag [The role of self-efficacy in influencing health behavior]. In A. P. Buunk, D. van Kreveld, & R. van der Vlist (Eds.), *Sociale psychologie en stereotypen, organisaties, gezondheid.* Den Haag: Vuga.

Locke, E. A., Saari, L. M., Shaw, K. N., & Latham, G. P. (1981). Goal setting and task performance: 1969-1980. *Psychological Bulletin, 90*(1), 125-152.

Maddux, J. E., Brawley, L., & Boykin, A. (1995). Self-efficacy and healthy behavior; prevention, promotion, and detection. In J. E. Maddux (Ed.), *Self-efficacy, adaptation and adjustment: Theory, research, and application.* New York: Plenum Press.

Maddux, J. E., & Lewis, J. (1995). Self-efficacy and adjustment; basic principles and issues. In J. E. Maddux (Ed.), *Self-efficacy, adaptation and adjustment: Theory, research, and application.* New York: Plenum Press.

Marlatt, G. A., & Gordon, J. R. (Eds.). (1985). *Relapse prevention: Maintenance strategies in the treatment of addictive behaviors.* New York: The Guilford Press.

Melamed, B. G., & Siegel, L. J. (1975). Reduction of anxiety in children facing hospitalisation and surgery by use of filmed modeling. *Journal of Consulting and Clinical Psychology, 43,* 511-521.

Oetker-Black, S. L., Teeters D. L., Cukr, P. L., & Rininger, S. A. (1997). Self-efficacy enhanced preoperative instruction. *AORN Journal, 66*(5), 854-862.

O'Leary, A. (1985). Self-efficacy and health. *Behavioral Research & Therapy, 23,* 437-451.

Ozer, E. M., & Bandura, A. (1990). Mechanisms governing empowerment effects: A self-efficacy analysis. *Journal of Personality and Social Psychology, 58*(3), 472-486.

Padgett, D. K. (1991). Correlates of self-efficacy beliefs among patients with non-insulin dependent diabetes mellitus in Zagreb, Yugoslavia. *Patient Education and Counseling, 18,* 139-147.

Padgett, D., Mumford, E., Hynes, M., & Carter, R. (1988). Meta-analysis of the effect of educational and psychosocial interventions on management of diabetes mellitus. *Journal of Clinical Epidemiology, 41*(10), 1007-1030.

Rosenstock, I. M. (1985). Understanding and enhancing patient compliance with diabetic regimens. *Diabetes Care, 8*(6), 610-616.

Schunk, D. H., & Carbonari, J. P. (1984). Self-Efficacy Models. In J. D. Matarazzo, J. H. Herd, N. Miller, & S. Weiss (Eds.), *Behavioral health: A handbook of health enhancement and disease prevention* (pp. 230-257). New York: Wiley.

Schunk, D. H. (1982). Effects of effort attributional feedback on children's perceived self-efficacy and achievement. *Journal of Educational Psychology, 74*(4), 548-556.

Strecher, V. J., DeVellis, B. M., Becker, M. H., & Rosenstock, I. M. (1986). The role of self-efficacy in achieving health behavior change. *Health Education Quarterly, 13*(1), 73-91.

Taal, E. (1995). *Self-efficacy, self-management and patient education in rheumatoïd arthritis.* Doctoral dissertation, Technical University Twente, Eburon, Delft, the Netherlands.

Tucker, S., Gross, D., Fogg, L., Delaney, K., & Lapporte, R. (1998). The long-term efficacy of a behavioral parent training intervention for families with 2-year-olds. *Research in Nursing & Health, 21,* 199-210.

Visser, A. P., Spijker A .J., Smelt H., & Van der Kar A. G. A.(1994). Persoonlijke effectiviteit en de zelfzorg bij diabetespatiënten [Self-efficacy and self-care in patients with diabetes]. *European Association of Diabetes Educators Nieuwsbrief, 5*(2), 4-8.

Vries, H. de (1993). Determinanten van gedrag [Determinants of behavior]. In V. Damoiseaux, H. T. van der Molen, & G. J. Kok (Eds.), *Gezondheidsvoorlichting en gedragsverandering.* Assen, the Netherlands: Van Gorcum.

Wing, R. R., Epstein, L. H., Nowalk, M. P., Koeske, R., & Hagg, S. (1985). Behavior change, weight loss, and physiological improvements in type II diabetic patients. *Journal of Consulting and Clinical Psychology, 53*(1), 111-122.

# Part III

# Self-Efficacy and Other Clinical Conditions

# 7

# Self-Efficacy Targeted Treatments for Weight Loss in Postmenopausal Women

**Karen E. Dennis**
**Naomi Tomoyasu**
**Susan H. McCrone**
**Andrew P. Goldberg**
**Linda Bunyard**
**Bing Bing Qi**

The effectiveness of obesity treatment programs has improved in the last decade largely due to multi-faceted refinements (Brownell & Wadden, 1992) and longer interventions (Goodrick & Foreyt, 1991; Perri, Nezu, Patti, & McCann, 1989; Wadden & Bell, 1990). Nevertheless, epidemiological evidence indicates increased prevalence of obesity across time (Flegal, Carroll, Kuczmarski, & Johnson, 1998; Kuczmarski, Flegal, Campbell, & Johnson, 1994) and the persistence of obesity in nearly 34% of American women (Kuczmarski et al., 1994), rising with the individual's chronological age (Williamson, Kahn, Remington, & Anda, 1990). This increased prevalence of obesity despite improved treatments remains an unsolved paradox; hence, there is a quest to develop even more effective approaches for its treatment. Matching behavioral treatment programs to different types of obese clients is a rarely studied strategy, despite its inherent appeal. Thus, guidelines for identifying which individual might benefit most from which program remain elusive.

One widely promulgated but underinvestigated strategy involves matching individuals and programs according to the degree of overweight in an attempt to limit cost, risk, and intensity of approach (Brownell & Wadden, 1991). Another promising, yet underinvestigated, approach involves the targeted enhancement of self-efficacy. Self-efficacy, the belief in one's ability to successfully accomplish particular behaviors, is a major determinant of one's choice of activities, as well as the amount of effort and length of time expended in their pursuit (Bandura, 1977, 1997). Although several investigators have demonstrated positive relationships between self-efficacy and weight loss (Dennis & Goldberg, 1996; Edell, Edington, Herd, O'Brien, & Witkin, 1987; Jeffery et al., 1984), data were correlational. The theoretical underpinnings of self-efficacy have not been foundational to the design and evaluation of weight loss treatments.

Early studies of weight control that explored the role of self-efficacy tended to passively measure, rather than actively manipulate, this phenomenon. For example, positive associations between self-efficacy and weight loss have been observed during interventions (Bernier & Poser, 1984; Edell, Edington, Herd, O'Brien, & Witkin, 1987; Stotland & Zuroff, 1991; Strecher, DeVellis, Becker, & Rosenstock, 1986), and at 1-year and 2-year follow-ups (Jeffery et al., 1984). The few investigators who manipulated self-efficacy did so by changing attributions of weight loss from placebo to self (Chambliss & Murray, 1979), labeling successful weight loss behaviors as exceptional (Weinberg, Hughes, Critelli, England, & Jackson, 1984), and presenting cognitive-behavioral self-control strategies (Bernier & Poser, 1984). A research team which carried self-efficacy measurement briefly into the maintenance phase reported that self-efficacy was significantly related to weight loss, not during treatment, but 6 weeks and 6 months later (Bernier & Poser, 1984). More recently, and consistent with Social Cognitive Theory, studies also supported the bidirectionality of this relationship in that self-efficacy not only impacted weight loss but was affected by it (Clark, Cargill, Medieros, & Pera, 1996; Dennis & Goldberg, 1996; Pinto, Clark, Cruess, Szymanski, & Pera, 1999). None of these studies, however, used the theoretical dynamics posited to enhance self-efficacy to design weight loss treatments or test their effectiveness.

The four dynamics that Bandura asserted to enhance self-efficacy are performance accomplishments, vicarious experience, verbal persuasion, and emotional arousal (Bandura, 1977). Using these four dynamics in the treatment of obesity means integrating them within state-of-the-art weight-loss programs. Multifaceted behavioral approaches to obesity treatment involve increasingly sophisticated interventions. These approaches include:

1.  Behavioral techniques and cognitive strategies for goal setting, problem solving, cognitive restructuring, stress management, and self-efficacy;
2.  Nutrition education to incorporate healthy food choices and helpful eating behaviors; and
3.  Social support through group dynamics to enhance and use extant support networks (Brownell & Kramer, 1994; Foreyt & Poston, 1998; Wadden & Bell, 1990).

Moreover, the marked heterogeneity among obese individuals has led to the evolution of matching clients to treatments (Agras, 1991; Brownell & Wadden, 1991; Fitzgibbon & Kirschenbaum, 1990). One of the latest matching approaches involves the treatment of binge eating (Marcus, Wing, & Hopkins, 1988), yet distinguishing the obese binge eater from the non-binge eater (Rossiter & Agras, 1990) and structuring appropriate interventions (Telch, Agras, Rossiter, Wilfley, & Kenardy, 1990) is in the early stages of evolution. Moreover, a recent attempt to develop a behavioral taxonomy for obese women was not predictive of weight loss outcomes (Schlundt et al., 1991). Most interventions that match obesity treatments to heterogeneous clients emphasize the external features of treatment, such as professional versus lay-led groups, self-direction versus super-imposed structure, variations in the length of treatment (Brownell & Wadden, 1992; Goodrick & Foreyt, 1991), and very-low-calorie diets (Wadden, Sternberg, Letizia, Stunkard, & Foster, 1989; Wadden, Stunkard, & Liebschutz, 1988). Few target the internal belief structures of obese clients.

Most treatments for obesity also are not strongly grounded in a theoretical base (Wilson, 1994). For more than two decades of clinical practice and research, the behavioral treatment of obesity (versus pharmaceutical and surgical approaches, for example) has emanated from an array of well-established, as well as more evolutionary, psychological principles. These principles include behavior modification and knowledge building (Brownell & Fairburn, 1995; Brownell & Wadden, 1992; Wadden & VanItallie, 1992; Wilson, 1994), cognitive therapy (Akins, Hollandsworth, & Alcorn, 1983; Beck, 1995), and self-awareness (Cargill, Clark, Pera, Niaura, & Abrams, 1999; Webb, Marsh, Schneiderman, & Davis, 1989). There are few studies which deal with self-efficacy as a theoretical component of obesity treatment, rather than as a correlate of predictors or outcomes.

Unfortunately, self-efficacy theory often is tested when it exerts only a partial influence over the behavior of interest (Bandura, 1997), thus it often fails to emerge as a strong predictor. In the case of weight management, obesity results when energy intake exceeds energy expenditure, both of which are affected by a combination of behavioral, environmental, metabolic, and genetic factors. Although *both*, food intake and exercise, are modifiable behaviors, eating self-efficacy typically is the target of interest (Clark et al., 1996; Stotland & Zuroff, 1991), even when the major outcome variable is physical activity (Foreyt, Brunner, Goodrick, St. Jeor, & Miller, 1995).

In our previous studies of weight loss in obese women (Dennis & Goldberg, 1996), Q methodology identified two distinct types of weight control self-efficacy beliefs: Assureds and Disbelievers. The women categorized as Assureds reported significantly greater self-esteem and less depression than the Disbelievers and sought a significantly less stringent "ideal" body weight. At treatment termination both Assureds and Disbelievers lost a significant amount of weight, but the Assureds lost significantly more weight than the Disbelievers. Disbelievers who shifted to an Assured belief during treatment lost comparable weight to women who were Assured at treatment onset. Based on these results, we hypothesized that intrinsic belief systems, as categorized by Q methodology, are important determinants in the ability to lose weight and might serve as a pretreatment indicator of potential success. This study was designed to categorize the weight control self-efficacy beliefs of obese, postmenopausal women using Q methodology and to determine the effects of self-efficacy targeted interventions versus a structured, nutrition-oriented, but nontargeted treatment on weight loss outcomes.

## METHODS

### Sample

Postmenopausal women 50-65 years old were recruited by media advertising and referrals by providers and friends/family and then were screened by telephone to ascertain whether they met inclusion criteria for participation. Women were required to have a Body Mass Index (BMI) of 27 to 40 kg/m$^2$, which approximates 20%-60% over recommended body weight based on the midpoint, medium frame of the Metropolitan Life Insurance tables (Metropolitan Life Insurance & Company, 1983). Responses also had to indicate that women were without menses for one year, sedentary, nonsmoking, and with limited alcohol consumption. They also could not have metabolic, endocrine, cardiovascular, musculoskeletal, or renal disorders, or be on medications (especially estrogen, serotonin uptake inhibitors or antidepressants) that may impact on obesity and its behavioral treatment. Women who met these initial inclusion criteria were invited for a screening clinical visit in which informed consent was obtained as approved by the University of Maryland Institutional Review Board. Evaluation consisted of a medical examination, blood chemistries, and collection of questionnaires as previously described (Berman, Nicklas, Rogus, Dennis, & Goldberg, 1998).

### Treatment

The Weight Control Self-Efficacy Q sort (WCSEQ) categorized the self-efficacy belief of each woman as an Assured or Disbeliever as previously described (Dennis & Goldberg, 1996). The strongest positive correlation of each woman's Q sort with one of the existent factor arrays (Assured or Disbeliever) determined her self-efficacy type. Women were stratified by self-efficacy type and randomly assigned to one of three treatment groups: Assured Treatment (AT), Disbeliever Treatment (DT) or Non-targeted Treatment (NT). Assureds were randomly assigned to AT which specifically targeted the weight control self-efficacy beliefs of that type, or NT which served as a control group; Disbelievers were randomly assigned to DT which specifically targeted the weight control self-efficacy beliefs of that type, or NT (see Figure 7.1).

The multifaceted weight loss treatments included diet, low-intensity walking, and lifestyle behavioral change. The only treatment parameter that differed was the systematic approach to enhancing self-efficacy, with AT and DT compared to control (NT). Since the dietary instruction and walking components were identical among treatments, and all women received these components, they are described first, with differences between treatments detailed separately. All three types of treatments (AT, DT, NT) met weekly over the course of 6 months (24 weeks), in hour-long classroom sessions followed by a structured, 45-minute walking period. Groups, consisting of 15 women in each, were "closed" so that the same women consistently met together and with the same therapists.

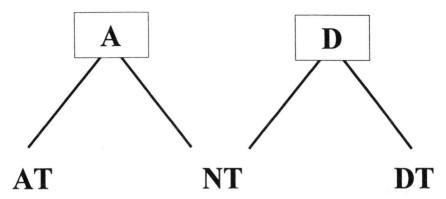

**Figure 7.1.** Schemata for randomization of Assureds (A) and Disbelievers (D) to Assured Treatment (AT), Nontargeted Treatment (NT), or Disbeliever Treatment (DT).

***Dietary Instruction and Low-Intensity Walking.*** The nontargeted, didactic dietary instruction followed NCEP recommendations (Expert Panel, 1993) with portions controlled so that intake was restricted by 300-500 calories per day to promote weight loss (WL) of approximately 0.5 kg/week. The use of the American Diabetic Association exchange system facilitated the selection of equivalent food items in accordance with individual preferences. Used with over 400 research participants of both genders and diverse ethnic groups across the age span in multiple research projects that address different research hypotheses this program consistently engenders an average of 8-9 kg WL in 6 months (Bunyard, Katzel, Busby-Whitehead, Wu, & Goldberg, 1998; Dengel, Katzel, & Goldberg, 1995; Dennis & Goldberg, 1996; Landkammer, Katzel, Engelhardt, Simpson, & Goldberg, 1992; Nicklas, Katzel, Bunyard, Dennis, & Goldberg, 1997). The dietitian was well versed in teaching a heart-healthy diet, blinded to assured or disbeliever status of the women, and held her instructions constant across all groups. Low-intensity walking was incorporated for its potential to facilitate dietary-induced weight loss, provide psychological uplift (Gavin, 1988), serve as an alternative activity to eating for emotional reasons, and enhance physiological benefits by reducing metabolic risk factors for cardiovascular disease (CVD). Women in all three treatment groups gradually increased their walking program until they reached 45 minutes three times a week at 50% of their $VO_2$ max.

***Self-Efficacy-Based Treatment.*** The objective of the targeted treatments was to directly affect self-efficacy, self-esteem, mood states, and eating behaviors to diminish food intake and increase physical activity, which lowers body weight and in turn affects CVD risk factors. AT and DT treatments were based on:

1. The four dynamics that Bandura (1977) identified as strengthening self-efficacy: performance accomplishment, vicarious experience, verbal persuasion, and emotional arousal, with the program content, tone, and delivery

tailored to meet the unique needs of the Assured and Disbeliever self-efficacy types;

2. The structure of the Assured or Disbeliever self-efficacy types elucidated by Q methodology; and

3. The self-esteem, mood, eating behaviors, and difficulty controlling overeating of the Assureds or Disbelievers found in our previous research (Dennis & Goldberg, 1996).

Targeted treatments were delivered by a nurse-psychologist team who met with all groups, and weekly with each other, to assure reliability of treatment implementation.

The goal of AT was to support and further strengthen the confident efficacy beliefs of the Assured type of obese women. Therapist-client and client-client interactions were characterized by the positive expectation that individuals are responsible for their weight management. The goal of DT was to build and instill confidence in Disbeliever women that they could successfully accomplish the behaviors needed for weight control, thereby converting women from the dependent Disbeliever to the Assured self-efficacy type. Different from the AT approach, DT was intensely structured and organized, using components of Social Learning Theory to help Disbelievers adopt characteristics of the Assured belief system.

***Nontargeted Treatment (Control).*** The interdisciplinary obesity research program uses a carefully structured, nutrition-oriented, behavioral weight loss intervention in multiple studies that address diverse hypotheses. This successful, 6-month didactic approach has enabled an average of 8 to 9 kg weight loss in both men and women (Coon, Bleecker, Drinkwater, Meyers, & Goldberg, 1989; Dennis, & Goldberg, 1993). In this study, nontargeted treatment (NT) followed the same diet and walking components as prescribed for AT and DT, but focused on nutrition and not targeted self-efficacy content. Weight loss activities, such as smaller portion sizes and adoption of traditional behavioral techniques, were encouraged and reinforced. Women understood that the goal for all groups was weight loss, and all women were encouraged and praised for their positive actions.

## Measures

Data were collected immediately prior to and at the completion of the interventions; the reliability and validity of the self-report questionnaires used in this study are well documented.

***Affective States and Eating Behaviors.*** Mood was measured by the Profile of Mood States (POMS; McNair, Lorr, & Droppleman, 1971). Depression was assessed more specifically by the Center for Epidemiologic Studies Depression Scale (CES-D; Radloff, 1977), since it does not contain items that reflect diminished intake or changes in eating patterns as symptoms of depression. The Coopersmith Self-Esteem Inventory (SEI; Coopersmith, 1981) evaluated self-esteem. The Eating Self-Efficacy Scale (ESES; Glynn & Ruderman, 1986) reflected difficulty in dealing with overeating due to negative emotions and social situational factors, while the Eating Behavior Inventory (O'Neil et al., 1979) measured eating behaviors conducive to weight loss. The Binge Eating Scale (BES; Gormally, Black, Daston, & Rardin, 1982) measures binge eating indicators: eating what is subjectively perceived as large amounts of food, and having feelings/cognitions such as guilt and fear of being unable to stop. Dietary intake was collected through 7-day food records. The dietitian individually reviewed these food records in detail with each woman, and analyzed them with Nutritionist Four® (N-Squared Computing, San Bruno, CA).

*Body Composition.* Height in centimeters was measured at baseline only. Weight in kilograms was measured at baseline and at each visit until termination of the study. The same standing scale was used throughout the study. Women were dressed in light indoor clothing without shoes. Body Mass Index (BMI) was calculated as (weight [in kilograms]/height [in meters]$^2$). The waist: hip ratio (WHR) was obtained by dividing the circumference of the waist, measured at the narrowest point superior to the hip, by the circumference of the hip, measured at the greatest gluteal protruberance. The waist and hip were measured twice at each data collection interval, and an average of the two measures was used in data analysis.

*Maximal Aerobic Capacity ($VO_2$ Max) and Daily Physical Activity.* $VO_2$ max was measured on the treadmill at a work rate set at approximately 75% of predicted maximal heart rate. Work rates increased in a stepwise manner during exercise, and $VO_2$, $CO_2$ production and respiratory exchange ratio were recorded every 30 seconds during the protocol. A valid $VO_2$ max satisfied two of the following three criteria:

1. A heart rate > 90% of age expected maximum;
2. A maximal respiratory exchange ratio > 1.10; and,
3. The plateau criterion wherein $VO_2$ changes < 2 ml/kg/min between the final two increases in work rate.

## Statistical Analysis

Data analysis proceeded in multiple phases using SPSS-PC (SPSS, Inc.). Initially, repeated measures analysis of variance (ANOVA) used self-efficacy type (Assureds vs. Disbelievers) as the between-groups factor and time as the repeated measure. In accordance with the random assignment pattern (Figure 7.1), separate repeated measures ANOVAs subsequently analyzed outcomes from Assureds in AT versus Assureds in NT, then Disbelievers in DT versus Disbelievers in NT. Finally, repeated measures ANOVAs analyzed outcomes from transitions in self-efficacy type (e.g., those who were Assured at pre- and posttreatment vs. Disbelievers who became Assureds with treatment). When baseline values were significantly different between groups, repeated measures analyses of covariance

(ANCOVA) was used in the format described above for ANOVAs, with the baseline value as the covariate. Posthoc independent $t$-tests were used to ascertain group and time differences when a significant ($p < .05$) $F$ statistic emerged. All data presented are mean ± standard deviation; $p$ was considered significant when $< 0.05$.

# RESULTS

## Sample and Attrition

There were 82 postmenopausal women who participated in the project, with 59 providing pre- and posttreatment data and 23 dropping out of the program. At baseline, women who dropped out of treatment weighed significantly more and had a significantly higher BMI than women who completed the program (see Table 7.1). Noncompleters were significantly more likely to be unmarried than those who completed (9.6% vs. 45.2%, $\chi^2 = 11.8$, $p < 0.05$), but there was no significant difference in educational status among the groups. Moreover, significantly more dropouts than completers were obese prior to adolescence (34.7% vs. 18.5%) than had become obese later in life (65.2% vs. 81.5%, $\chi^2 = 8.3$, $p < 0.05$). In terms of self-efficacy belief, 52/82 (63%) of the women who initially enrolled were Assureds and 30/82 (37%) were Disbelievers. Of the 23 women who dropped out, there was no difference in the attrition rates between the two self-efficacy types; 15/52 (29%) Assureds who started in the study eventually dropped out as did 8/30 (27%) of the enrolled Disbelievers. Attrition, however, was markedly different by treatment type. Significantly *more* Disbelievers dropped from DT (16.2%) than NT (2.6%), while significantly *fewer* Assureds dropped from AT (14.0%) than NT (23.1%) ($\chi^2 = 5.3$, $p < 0.05$).

**TABLE 7.1. Baseline Measures of Program Completers Versus Dropouts**

| Measure | Completers ($n = 59$) | Dropouts ($n = 23$) |
|---|---|---|
| Age | 59.9 ± 5.7 | 59.7 ± 4.5 |
| Height | 158.3 ± 18.6 | 163.4 ± 6.9 |
| Weight (kg) | 86.1 ± 12.7 | 94.0 ± 14.1* |
| BMI (kg/m$^2$) | 32.8 ± 4.7 | 35.5 ± 4.4* |
| Waist (cm) | 94.6 ± 10.1 | 101.2 ± 11.0 |
| Hip (cm) | 116.5 ± 11.5 | 119.4 ± 11.2 |
| WHR | 0.81 ± 0.07 | 0.85 ± 0.08 |

*Note.* BMI = Body Mass Index; WHR = Waist:Hip Ratio.
*$p < .05$.

### TABLE 7.2. Baseline Measures of Assureds and Disbelievers

| Measure | Assureds ($n = 37$) | | Disbelievers ($n = 22$) | |
|---|---|---|---|---|
| Weight (kg) | 84.2 | ± 13.0 | 89.4 | ± 11.9 |
| BMI (kg/m$^2$) | 31.9 | ± 4.5 | 34.4 | ± 4.9 |
| Waist (cm) | 92.4 | ± 9.0 | 99.9 | ± 11.1* |
| Hip (cm) | 113.5 | ± 9.8 | 109.3 | ± 10.7* |
| WHR | 0.82 | ± 0.08 | 0.82 | ± 0.05 |
| VO$_2$ Max (L/min) | 1.6 | ± 0.2 | 1.7 | ± 0.3 |
| Depression[a] | 4.8 | ± 5.0 | 5.4 | ± 3.6 |
| Self-esteem[b] | 84.7 | ± 11.9 | 71.5 | ± 15.7** |
| Eating Behavior Inventory[b] | 75.6 | ± 8.5 | 70.2 | ± 8.1 |
| Binge Eating[a] | 11.5 | ± 6.6 | 19.4 | ± 9.6** |
| Difficulty Controlling Affect Overeating[a] | 62.3 | ± 21.5 | 74.4 | ± 20.4* |
| Difficulty Controlling Social Overeating[a] | 45.5 | ± 10.2 | 47.3 | ± 9.1 |

*Note.* BMI = Body Mass Index; WHR = Waist:Hip Ratio; L/min = liters/minute.
[a]Lower scores are better. [b]Higher scores are better.
*$p < .05$, **$p < .01$.

## Assureds and Disbelievers

At baseline there were 37 Assureds and 22 Disbelievers. Although the 5.2 kg difference in body weight was not significant, the Assureds had significantly smaller waist and hip circumferences (see Table 7.2). Behaviorally, the Assureds reported significantly less difficulty controlling overeating with negative affect, less binge eating symptomatology, and greater self esteem than the Disbelievers. After weight loss, the only significant difference between Assureds and Disbelievers on any of the measured variables was waist circumference (89.2 ± 10.1 cm Assureds vs. 96.1 ± 11.1 cm Disbelievers, $p < 0.05$).

## Treatment Effects

*Assureds.* There were no significant differences at baseline between Assureds in AT versus NT, indicating effectiveness of the randomization scheme. When weight loss outcomes were analyzed by pretreatment self-efficacy type, the Assureds in AT and the Assureds in NT fared equally well (see Table 7.3). There were significant differences from pre- to posttreatment for both treatment groups, but not between them. With treatment, the Assureds in AT lost 6.1 kg (7% of initial body weight) while the Assureds in NT lost 7.5 kg (9% of initial body weight).

**TABLE 7.3. Measures of Assureds in Assured (AT) Versus Nontargeted (NT) Treatment**

| Measure | Assureds in AT ($n = 20$) | | Assureds in NT ($n = 17$) | |
|---|---|---|---|---|
| | Baseline | Post weight loss | Baseline | Post weight loss |
| Weight (kg) | 86.1 ± 12.9 | 80.0 ± 14.9*** | 81.9 ± 13.0 | 74.4 ± 12.8*** |
| BMI (kg/m$^2$) | 32.6 ± 4.1 | 30.3 ± 4.9*** | 31.1 ± 5.0 | 28.1 ± 4.8*** |
| Waist (cm) | 93.4 ± 8.5 | 90.1 ± 9.6* | 91.2 ± 9.6 | 88.1 ± 10.9** |
| Hip (cm) | 114.9 ± 10.2 | 110.7 ± 11.2*** | 111.9 ± 9.5 | 107.8 ± 10.3** |
| WHR | 0.82 ± 0.08 | 0.82 ± 0.05 | 0.82 ± 0.07 | 0.82 ± 0.07 |
| VO$_2$ Max (L/min) | 1.6 ± 0.2 | 1.7 ± 0.2* | 1.6 ± 0.3 | 1.8 ± 0.3*** |
| Depression[a] | 4.6 ± 4.6 | 6.6 ± 6.1 | 5.1 ± 6.1 | 8.5 ± 7.4 |
| Self Esteem[b] | 85.0 ± 14.6 | 83.8 ± 12.5 | 84.3 ± 7.9 | 78.5 ± 11.0 |
| Eating Behavior Inventory[b] | 75.1 ± 8.8 | 85.5 ± 10.7*** | 76.8 ± 8.3 | 92.4 ± 6.1**† |
| Binge Eating[a] | 11.7 ± 7.6 | 10.4 ± 5.9 | 11.2 ± 5.5 | 7.5 ± 4.4** |
| Difficulty Controlling Affect Overeating[a] | 66.0 ± 20.8 | 60.5 ± 21.3 | 54.1 ± 22.1 | 43.9 ± 16.6† |
| Difficulty Controlling Social Overeating[a] | 45.2 ± 10.4 | 40.7 ± 9.7 | 46.3 ± 10.3 | 36.9 ± 11.0 |

*Note.* BMI = Body Mass Index; WHR = Waist:Hip Ratio; L/min = liters/minute.
[a]Lower scores are better. [b]Higher scores are better.
*$p < 0.05$, **$p < .01$, ***$p < .001$ baseline to post weight loss.
† $p < .05$ at baseline or at post weight loss between assureds in AT vs. NT.

Changes in other body habitus parameters reflect these equivalent decrements in body weight. There were no differences in VO$_2$ max or the increase in VO$_2$ max between Assureds in AT and NT. There were no significant differences between Assureds in AT versus NT on any affect measure. Significant differences in eating behaviors were limited and without pattern. Assureds in AT reported significantly less difficulty controlling overeating during negative affect, but paradoxically used significantly fewer eating behaviors conducive to weight loss.

***Disbelievers.*** There were no differences on any of the variables at pretreatment between Disbelievers in DT versus NT (Table 7.4). As seen with the Assureds, differences occurred from pre- to posttreatment rather than between treatment types. With treatment, the Disbelievers in DT lost 6.5 kg (7% of initial body weight), while the Disbelievers in NT lost 8.6 kg (10% of initial body weight) with concomitant decreases in other body habitus parameters. There were no differences in VO$_2$ max or the increase in VO$_2$ max between Disbelievers in DT and NT. There were no significant differences at posttreatment between Disbelievers in DT versus NT on any affect measure, although DT women had significantly less difficulty controlling overeating in socially acceptable circumstances than NT women.

**TABLE 7.4. Measures of Disbelievers in Disbeliever (DT) Versus Nontargeted (NT) Treatment**

| Measure | Disbelievers in DT (*n* = 10) | | Disbelievers in NT (*n* = 12) | |
|---|---|---|---|---|
| | Baseline | Post-weight loss | Baseline | Post-weight loss |
| Weight (kg) | 89.5 ± 11.8 | 83.0 ± 12.0** | 89.2 ± 12.5 | 80.6 ±11.0** |
| BMI (kg/m²) | 35.7 ± 4.2 | 32.8 ± 5.2** | 33.5 ± 5.4 | 30.6 ± 3.5* |
| Waist (cm) | 102.9 ± 14.4 | 97.5 ± 15.9* | 98.1 ± 8.9 | 95.3 ± 7.8 |
| Hip (cm) | 124.1 ± 10.8 | 118.2 ± 13.2* | 120.0 ± 10.8 | 112.8 ± 9.9** |
| WHR | 0.83± 0.04 | 0.84± 0.06 | 0.85± 0.06 | 0.82± 0.04 |
| VO₂ Max (L/mins) | 1.8 ± 0.2 | 1.9 ± 0.3* | 1.6 ± 0.3 | 1.7 ± 0.3* |
| Depression[a] | 6.1 ± 3.8 | 8.7 ± 7.5 | 4.7 ± 3.6 | 11.4 ± 9.7 |
| Self-esteem[b] | 74.7 ± 16.5 | 75.3 ± 15.7 | 69.6 ± 15.8 | 73.6 ±19.7 |
| Eating Behavior Inventory[b] | 70.0 ± 6.3 | 81.1 ± 7.9** | 70.4 ± 10.1 | 89.4 ± 8.9** |
| Binge Eating[a] | 21.8 ± 11.1 | 17.8 ± 8.3 | 17.8 ± 8.8 | 10.9 ± 8.2* |
| Difficulty Controlling Affect Overeating[a] | 78.7 ± 17.4 | 57.1 ± 23.7 | 70.1 ± 23.5 | 50.3 ±16.7* |
| Difficulty Controlling Social Overeating[a] | 47.6 ± 5.5 | 46.3 ± 5.6 | 47.1 ± 12.1 | 34.7 ± 4.6*†† |

*Note.* BMI = Body Mass Index; WHR = Waist:Hip Ratio; L/min = liters/minute.
[a]Lower scores are better. [b]Higher scores are better.
*$p < 0.05$, **$p < .01$, ***$p < .001$ baseline to postweight loss.
†† $p < .01$ at baseline or at postweight loss between disbelievers in DT vs. NT.

***Transitions in Self-Efficacy Types.*** Missing posttreatment Q sort data on 14 women affected the analysis of transitions in self-efficacy types. Of the 45 women who provided complete posttreatment data, all but one of the 27 Assureds retained their Assured weight control self-efficacy belief at the end of the weight loss program. Thus, differences between Assureds who remained Assureds and those who became Disbelievers could not be analyzed. Of the 17 Disbelievers for whom posttreatment Q sort data were available, 10 transitioned to Assureds while 7 retained their Disbeliever stance. There were equivalent numbers of Disbelievers in DT and NT who made the transition to an Assured self-efficacy belief. There was equivalent weight loss during treatment and no other significant differences in affect or eating behaviors. Those who continued to be Disbelievers at posttreatment reported significantly greater symptoms of depression (CES-D) (16.2 ± 11.3 vs. 6.7 ± 3.8, $p < .05$). Although not significantly different, Disbelievers who became Assureds reported less binge eating symptomatology and less difficulty controlling overeating with negative affect, as well as greater use of eating behaviors conducive to weight loss. In terms of affect, Disbelievers who became Assureds reported less tension, fatigue, and trait anxiety, and greater vigor than those who remained Disbelievers. Data are not shown, but follow patterns similar to those shown in Table 7.2.

## DISCUSSION

Results of this study support the incorporation of self-efficacy enhancement in the behavioral treatment of obesity. Viewed from the measures of body habitus as well as affect and eating behaviors, there were some significant differences between Assureds and Disbelievers at baseline. Significantly greater waist and hip measurements in the Disbelievers were reflected in greater weight and BMI. Similar to our previous findings (Dennis & Goldberg, 1996), at baseline the Assureds reported significantly greater self-esteem, fewer symptoms of binge eating, and less difficulty controlling overeating at times of negative affect than the Disbelievers. Improvement in these variables with weight loss for the Disbelievers erased significant differences between them and the Assureds.

More cogent, however, are the results of the Assureds in AT versus NT and the Disbelievers in DT versus NT. Data from Disbelievers in DT versus NT support the adoption of our NT for these women, realizing that the small number of women in Disbeliever groups adversely impacted statistical power. Nevertheless, Disbelievers in NT made statistically significant improvements in their use of eating behaviors conducive to weight loss, binge eating symptoms, and difficulty controlling their overeating during times of negative affect and in various social situations. Moreover, Disbelievers' attrition rate from NT was significantly less than from DT.

It is noteworthy that our NT is didactic rather than small-group facilitative. While AT and DT deliberately sought to increase self-efficacy through their targeted theory-based structure and focus on cognitive, behavioral, and emotional strategies, NT likely increased self-efficacy through the performance accomplishment and verbal persuasion that are inherent in these rigorous, didactic sessions for dietary change. The dietitian did not target the self-efficacy type, but she rigorously taught the dietary information and exacted compliance in following course instruction and maintaining daily food records. Thus, the highly-structured, precisely-monitored approach of NT may have met Disbelievers' wavering self-efficacy beliefs and dependency needs more than did the DT approach that tried to lead them to greater independence and an Assured belief type by treatment termination.

Among the Assureds, there were too few significant differences in outcomes between AT and NT to argue the differential effectiveness of one treatment type over another. Significant differences in body habitus and $VO_2$ max occurred across time rather than between groups. The significantly greater use of eating behaviors conducive to weight loss found in the usual care group (NT) may reflect the greater emphasis on dietary habits that was inherent in that treatment. Differential attrition, however, once again emerged as a best-practice marker. Despite the lack of significant differences in outcome variables, Assureds were observably different from Disbelievers during treatment. Monitoring food intake was encouraged for its known contribution to successful weight loss, but individuality in acceptance of this responsibility was the focus. It may have been that didactic NT was too confining for the Assureds with their stronger self-efficacy beliefs, causing more of them to drop out of NT than AT.

The overall attrition rate of 28% is comparable to other weight loss studies of this treatment length (Clark, Guise, & Niaura, 1995). One of the most striking differences between treatment types, however, was attrition rate, with significantly more Assureds dropping from NT than AT and significantly more Disbelievers dropping from DT than NT. Treatment delivery type may have influenced attrition rate, since NT was more highly structured than either AT or DT. Disbelievers may need a rigid structure and thus will continue to pursue a program that meets their needs, while Assureds may need the greater flexibility found in AT. Firm structure versus flexibility has been posited as a way to target obesity treatments to different clients' needs (Brownell & Wadden, 1991). Unfortunately, to our knowledge, no studies have examined this hypothesis. While it is clear that self-efficacy type is not the same phenomenon as preference for type of treatment structure, the two constructs seem to be associated. Thus, self-efficacy type may serve as a means to identify different types of treatment needs among postmenopausal women. Because longer treatments seem to lead to greater weight loss (Brownell & Kramer, 1994; Goodrick & Foreyt, 1991; Wadden & Bell, 1990), keeping women in treatment for the duration of the program should lead to improved outcomes for more of them.

In this study, NT and DT were equivalent in their ability to help Disbeliever women transition to an Assured self-efficacy type. As we found in our previous research (Dennis & Goldberg, 1996) Disbelievers who became Assureds during the course of treatment were more similar to the women who were always Assureds than they were to Disbelievers who remained Disbelievers. Weight loss was equivalent whether or not Disbeliever women became Assured, but those who transitioned did have improved affect and eating behaviors. Low statistical power likely afffected statistical significance in this small number of women (10 Disbelievers who transitioned to Assured vs. 7 who did not), but data are promising and results reflect the expected direction.

In AT, DT, and NT, reduction in body weight and improvements in other behavioral variables were similar for Assureds and Disbelievers. Moreover, both targeted and nontargeted treatments were equivalent in their ability to help Disbeliever women transition to an Assured self-efficacy type. It appears that performance accomplishment in weight loss overrode all treatment approaches in enhancing self-efficacy and seemed to be the most important dynamic in this treatment program. Thus, weight loss was its own very strong reinforcement. The preeminence of performance accomplishment in enhancing self-efficacy is consistent with the earliest (Bandura, 1977) as well as more recent versions of Social Learning Theory (Bandura, 1997). In addition, findings are consistent with significant improvements in eating self-efficacy after only 12 weeks of treatment (Pinto, Clark, Cruess, Szymanski, & Pera, 1999) and with those for participants of a 26-week very-low-calorie dietary program (Clark, Cargill, Medieros, & Pera, 1996). The successful weight loss, change in eating behaviors, and increase in physical conditioning that women in all groups achieved argues for the incorporation of strategies to enhance self-efficacy but not for the need for targeted treatments based on self-efficacy type.

# REFERENCES

Agras, S. (1991). *Overweight people are not all the same: Matching types and treatments.* Paper presented at the Society of Behavioral Medicine: Twelfth Annual Scientific Sessions, Washington, DC.

Akins, T., Hollandsworth, J. G., Jr., & Alcorn, J. D. (1983). Visual and verbal modes of information processing and cognitively-based coping strategies: An extension and replication. *Behaviour Research and Therapy, 21*(1), 69-73.

Bandura, A. (1977). Self-efficacy: Toward a unifying theory of behavioral change. *Psychological Review, 84*(2), 191-215.

Bandura, A. (1997). *Self-efficacy: The exercise of control.* New York: W. H. Freeman.

Beck, J. S. (1995). *Cognitive therapy: Basics and beyond.* New York: Guilford.

Berman, D. M., Nicklas, B. J., Rogus, E. M., Dennis, K. E., & Goldberg, A. P. (1998). Regional differences in adrenoceptor binding and fat cell lipolysis in obese, postmenopausal women. *Metabolism, 47*(4), 467-473.

Bernier, M., & Poser, E. G. (1984). The relationship between self-efficacy, attributions, and weight loss in a weight rehabilitation program. *Rehabilitation Psychology, 29*(2), 95-105.

Brownell, K. D., & Fairburn, C. G. (1995). *Eating disorders and obesity: A comprehensive handbook* (1st ed.). New York: Guilford.

Brownell, K. D., & Kramer, F. M. (1994). Behavioral management of obesity. In G. L. Blackburn & B. S. Kanders (Eds.), *Obesity: Pathophysiology, Psychology and Treatment* (pp. 231-252). New York: Chapman & Hall.

Brownell, K. D., & Wadden, T. A. (1991). The heterogeneity of obesity: Fitting treatments to individuals. *Behavior Therapy, 22,* 153-177.

Brownell, K. D., & Wadden, T. A. (1992). Etiology and treatment of obesity: Understanding a serious, prevalent, and refractory disorder. *Journal of Consulting and Clinical Psychology, 60*(4), 505-517.

Bunyard, L. B., Katzel, L. I., Busby-Whitehead, M. J., Wu, Z., & Goldberg, A. P. (1998). Energy requirements of middle-aged men are modifiable by physical activity. *American Journal of Clinical Nutrition, 68,* 1136-1142.

Cargill, B. R., Clark, M. M., Pera, V., Niaura, R. S., & Abrams, D. B. (1999). Binge eating, body image, depression, and self-efficacy in an obese clinical population. *Obesity Research, 7*(4), 379-386.

Chambliss, C. A., & Murray, E. J. (1979). Efficacy attribution, locus of control, and weight loss. *Cognitive Therapy and Research, 3*(4), 349-353.

Clark, M. M., Cargill, B. R., Medieros, M. L., & Pera, V. (1996). Changes in self-efficacy following obesity treatment. *Obesity Research, 4,* 179-181.

Clark, M. M., Guise, B. J., & Niaura, R. S. (1995). Obesity level and attrition: Support for patient-treatment matching in obesity treatment. *Obesity Research, 3*(1), 63-64.

Coon, P. J., Bleecker, E. R., Drinkwater, D. T., Meyers, D. A., & Goldberg, A. P. (1989). Effects of body composition and exercise capacity on glucose tolerance, insulin, and lipoprotein lipids in healthy older men: A cross-sectional and longitudinal intervention study. *Metabolism, 38*(12), 1201-1209.

Coopersmith, S. (1981). *Self-esteem inventories.* Palo Alto, CA: Consulting Psychologists Press.

Dengel, J. L., Katzel, L. I., & Goldberg, A. P. (1995). Effect of an American Heart Association diet, with or without weight loss, on lipids in obese middle-aged and older men. *American Journal of Clinical Nutrition, 62,* 715-721.

Dennis, K. E., & Goldberg, A. P. (1993). Differential effects of body fatness and body fat distribution on risk factors for cardiovascular disease in women: Impact of weight loss. *Arteriosclerosis and Thrombosis, 13,* 1487-1494.

Dennis, K. E., & Goldberg, A. P. (1996). Weight control self-efficacy types and positive transitions affect weight loss in obese women. *Addictive Behaviors, 21*(1), 103-116.

Edell, B. H., Edington, S., Herd, B., O'Brien, R. M., & Witkin, G. (1987). Self-efficacy and self-motivation as predictors of weight loss. *Addictive Behaviors, 12,* 63-66.

Expert Panel. (1993). The National Cholesterol Education (NCEP) expert panel on detection, evaluation, and treatment of high blood cholesterol/adult treatment panel/summary of the second report. *Journal of the American Medical Association, 269,* 3015-3023.

Fitzgibbon, M. L., & Kirschenbaum, D. S. (1990). Heterogeneity of clinical presentation among obese individuals seeking treatment. *Addictive Behaviors, 15*(3), 291-295.

Flegal, K. M., Carroll, M. D., Kuczmarski, R. J., & Johnson, C. L. (1998). Overweight and obesity in the United States: Prevalence and trends, 1960-1994. *International Journal of Obesity, 22,* 39-47.

Foreyt, J. P., Brunner, R. L., Goodrick, K., St. Jeor, S., & Miller, G. D. (1995). Psychological correlates of reported physical activity in normal-weight and obese adults: The Reno diet-heart study. *International Journal of Obesity, 19*(Suppl. 4), 69-72.

Foreyt, J. P., & Poston, W. S. C. (1998). What is the role of cognitive-behavior therapy in patient management? *Obesity Research, 6*(Suppl. 1), 18-22.

Gavin, J. (1988). Psychological issues in exercise prescription. *Sports Medicine, 6,* 1-10.

Glynn, S. M., & Ruderman, A. J. (1986). The development and validation of an Eating Self Efficacy Scale. *Cognitive Therapy and Research, 10*(4), 403-420.

Goodrick, G. K., & Foreyt, J. P. (1991). Why treatments for obesity don't last. *Journal of the American Dietetic Association, 91,* 1243-1247.

Gormally, J., Black, S., Daston, S., & Rardin, D. (1982). The assessment of binge eating severity among obese persons. *Addictive Behaviors, 7,* 47-55.

Jeffery, R. W., Bjornson-Benson, W. M., Rosenthal, B. S., Lindquist, R. A., Kurth, C. L., & Johnson, S. L. (1984). Correlates of weight loss and its maintenance over two years of follow-up among middle-aged men. *Preventive Medicine, 13,* 155-168.

Kuczmarski, R. J., Flegal, K. M., Campbell, S. M., & Johnson, C. L. (1994). Increasing prevalence of overweight among US adults: The National Health and Nutrition Examination Surveys, 1960 to 1991. *Journal of the American Medical Association, 272*(3), 206-211.

Landkammer, J., Katzel, L., Engelhardt, S., Simpson, K., & Goldberg, A. (1992). Cardiovascular risk factors modification after dietary therapy of obese older men. *Gerontologist, 32,* 71A.

Marcus, M. D., Wing, R. R., & Hopkins, J. (1988). Obese binge eaters: Affect, cognitions, and response to behavioral weight control. *Journal of Consulting and Clinical Psychology, 56,* 433-439.

McNair, D. M., Lorr, M., & Droppleman, L. F. (1971). *EITS Manual for the Profile of Mood States*. San Diego, CA: Educational and Industrial Testing Service.

Metropolitan Life Insurance Company. (1983). 1983 Metropolitan height and weight tables. *Statistical Bulletin of the Metropolitan Life Insurance Company, 64,* 2-4.

Nicklas, B. J., Katzel, L. I., Bunyard, L. B., Dennis, K. E., & Goldberg, A. P. (1997). Effects of an American Heart Association diet and weight loss on lipoprotein lipids in obese, postmenopausal women. *American Journal of Clinical Nutrition, 66,* 853-859.

O'Neil, P. M., Currey, H. S., Hirsch, A. A., Malcolm, R. J., Sexauer, J. D., Riddle, F. E., & Taylor, C. I. (1979). Development and validation of the Eating Behavior Inventory. *Journal of Behavioral Assessment, 1*(2), 123-132.

Perri, M. G., Nezu, A. M., Patti, E. T., & McCann, K. L. (1989). Effect of length of treatment on weight loss. *Journal of Consulting and Clinical Psychology, 57,* 450-452.

Pinto, B. M., Clark, M. M., Cruess, D. G., Szymanski, L., & Pera, V. (1999). Changes in self-efficacy and decisional balance for exercise among obese women in a weight management program. *Obesity Research, 7*(3), 288-292.

Radloff, L. S. (1977). The CES-D Scale: A self-report depression scale for research in the general population. *Applied Psychological Measurement, 1*(3), 385-401.

Rossiter, E. M., & Agras, W. S. (1990). An empirical test of the DSM-III-R definition of binge. *International Journal of Eating Disorders, 9*(5), 513-518.

Schlundt, D. G., Taylor, D., Hill, J. O., Sbrocco, T., Pope-Cordle, J., Kasser, T., & Arnold, D. (1991). A behavioral taxonomy of obese female participants in a weight-loss program. *American Journal of Clinical Nutrition, 53*(5), 1151-1158.

Stotland, S., & Zuroff, D. C. (1991). Relations between multiple measures of dieting self-efficacy and weight change in a behavioral weight control program. *Behavior Therapy, 22,* 47-59.

Strecher, V. J., DeVellis, B. M., Becker, M. H., & Rosenstock, I. M. (1986). The role of self-efficacy in achieving health behavior change. *Health Education Quarterly, 13*(1), 73-91.

Telch, C. F., Agras, W. S., Rossiter, E. M., Wilfley, D., & Kenardy, J. (1990). Group cognitive-behavioral treatment for the nonpurging bulimic: An initial evaluation. *Journal of Consulting and Clinical Psychology, 58,* 629-635.

Wadden, T. A., & Bell, S. T. (1990). Obesity. In A. S. Bellack, M. Hersen, & A. E. Kazdin (Eds.), *International handbook of behavior modification and therapy* (2nd ed., pp. 449-473). New York: Plenum.

Wadden, T. A., Sternberg, J. A., Letizia, K. A., Stunkard, A. J., & Foster, G. D. (1989). Treatment of obesity by very low calorie diet, behavior therapy, and their combination: a five-year perspective. *International Journal of Obesity, 13*(Suppl. 2), 39-46.

Wadden, T. A., Stunkard, A. J., & Liebschutz, J. (1988). Three year follow-up of the treatment of obesity by very-low-calorie diet, behavior therapy, and their combination. *Journal of Consulting and Clinical Psychology, 56,* 925-928.

Wadden, T. A., & VanItallie, T. B. (1992). *Treatment of the seriously obese patient* (1st ed.). New York: Guilford.

Webb, W. M., Marsh, K. L., Schneiderman, W., & Davis, B. (1989). Interaction between self-monitoring and manipulated states of self-awareness. *Journal of Personality and Social Psychology, 56*(1), 70-80.

Weinberg, R. S., Hughes, H. H., Critelli, J. W., England, R., & Jackson, A. (1984). Effects of preexisting and manipulated self-efficacy on weight loss in a self-control program. *Journal of Research in Personality, 18,* 352-358.

Williamson, D. F., Kahn, H. S., Remington, P. L., & Anda, R. F. (1990). The 10-year incidence of overweight and major weight gain in US adults. *Archives of Internal Medicine, 150,* 665-672.

Wilson, G. T. (1994). Behavioral treatment of obesity: Thirty years and counting. *Advances in Behavioral Research Therapy, 16,* 31-75.

# 8

# An Intervention to Increase Quality of Life and Self-Care Self-Efficacy and Decrease Symptoms in Breast Cancer Patients

Elise L. Lev
Karen M. Daley
Norma E. Conner
Margaret Reith
Cristina Fernandez
Steven V. Owen

Medical treatments for patients with chronic illnesses are increasingly being evaluated by quality of life issues as well as life extension (Andrykowski et al., 1995; Del Giudice, Leszcz, Pritchard, Vincent, & Goodwin, 1997; Ferrell et al., 1996). As the effectiveness of antineoplastic agents became widely known, many new antineoplastic drugs were introduced in the 1980s and concern about patient quality of life increased (Cella et al., 1993). Measures of quality of life may include health functioning, socioeconomic, psychological and family concerns, physical symptoms, psychological symptoms, well-being, and social support, symptom distress, and the impact of symptoms on activities (Ferrans, 1990; Ferrell, Wisdom, Wenzl, & Brown, 1989; Longman, Braden, & Mishel, 1996).

Uncontrolled side effects of treatment, including anticipatory nausea and vomiting and weight gain, are problems for women receiving chemotherapy for breast cancer that may decrease quality of life and potentially threaten survival (Del Giudice, Leszcz, Pritchard, Vincent, & Goodwin, 1997; Demark-Wahnefried, Winer, & Rimer, 1993; Longman, Braden, & Mishel, 1996). Although follow-up studies reported that distress may persist over time, patients receiving chemotherapy took few preventive actions to manage side effects of treatment (Dodd, 1984; Longman, Braden, & Mishel, 1996).

Attention to psychosocial issues is an integral part of a comprehensive oncologic program (Coluzzi et al., 1995). Psychological interventions to enhance quality of life and given to cancer patients early in the adjustment process may be important for reducing emotional distress, enhancing coping and improving adjustment (Andersen, 1992; Baider, Uziely, & DeNour, 1994; Cunningham, Edmonds, & Williams, 1999; Del Giudice, Leszcz, Pritchard, Vincent, & Goodwin, 1997; Fawzy, 1995; Fawzy, Fawzy, Arndt, & Pasnau, 1995; Walker & Eremin, 1996). Treatment components underlying different studies included the use of various behavior therapy procedures such as relaxation training, cognitive distraction, and goal setting (Burish, 1994; Edgar, Rosberger, & Nowlis, 1992; Edmonds, Lockwood, & Cunningham, 1999; Fawzy & Fawzy, 1994; Vasterling, Jenkins, Tope, & Burish, 1993; Walker et al., 1999). Studies investigated effects of interventions given by trained intervenors to newly diagnosed adult cancer patients. When interventions were delivered on five occasions, significant differences in outcomes were found (Burish, Synder, & Jenkins, 1991; Edgar, Rosberger, & Nowlis, 1992; Vasterling, Jenkins, Tope, & Burish, 1993). Behavioral interventions for coping with and minimizing aversive reactions to cancer chemotherapy were used to teach coping skills, resulting in decreased side effects and improved emotional coping (Burish, 1994; Edgar, Rosberger, & Nowlis, 1992; Vasterling, Jenkins, Tope, & Burish, 1993). Edgar, Rosberger, and Nowlis (1992) analyzed outcomes of patients with breast cancer ($n = 98$) and reported that there was a significant decrease in distress after the intervention, followed by improved emotional coping during the following year; a weakness of the study was the absence of a control group.

Orem (1995) defined self-care as actions that regulate one's functioning in the interests of one's life, integrated functioning, and well-being and noted that a single self-care practice is therapeutic to the degree that it actually contributes to the regulation or control of disease processes. Self-care strategies decrease anxiety and stress symptoms, and result in decreased morbidity (Dodd, 1984; Lev, 1992). Self-care requirements arise not only from disease but also from medical care measures prescribed by physicians. Cancer patients' self-care activities have been used to manage side effects, decrease anxiety and stress symptoms, the disease process, and control or avoid symptoms (Dodd, 1984). Determining self-care behaviors that constitute a positive response to cancer chemotherapy supports Orem's (1995) recommendation to determine which self-care behaviors constitute a therapeutic response.


## SELF-EFFICACY


Self-efficacy theory (Bandura, 1997) provides a framework for a specific supportive educative intervention that enables people to develop their self-care behaviors and provides a comprehensive analysis of determinants of behavior change. Bandura (1997) noted that perceived self-efficacy mediates health behaviors because people need to believe they can master and adhere to health-promoting habits in order to devote the effort necessary to succeed. Belief in one's competence to perform self-care (self-efficacy) must occur before self-care can be attempted.

Research has demonstrated that measurements of perceived self-efficacy do not change with repeated testing in the absence of interventions and that understanding of patients' self-management behaviors is improved when efficacy perceptions are taken into account (Beck & Lund, 1981). Stress reduction effects are explained more by a person's perceived self-efficacy than by direct behavioral reduction of stress (Bandura, 1997). Efficacy expectations, formed through information derived from four primary sources, are listed in order of their hypothesized power: actual performance accomplishments, vicarious experience, verbal persuasion, and physiological states (Bandura, 1997).

Perceptions of self-efficacy predicted intention to quit smoking, increased patients' participation in cancer screening programs, and increased patients' adjustment to cancer diagnosis (Lev, 1997; Lev, Paul, & Owen, 1999). Perceptions of self-efficacy were correlated with quality of life and depression at 1 and 6 months after stroke (Robinson-Smith, Johnston, & Allen, 2000). Education for self-efficacy was shown to have prolonged benefits in health conditions (Bandura, 1997; Cunningham, Lockwood, & Cunningham, 1991; Lorig, Mazonson, & Holman, 1993). Without intervention, cancer patients' measures of self-care self-efficacy and adjustment decreased over time (Lev, Paul, & Owen, 1999). Carey and Burish (1988) suggested that effective psychosocial interventions given to cancer patients may increase cancer patients' self-efficacy; however, previous studies of interventions for cancer patients had not measured patients' self-efficacy.

## EFFICACY-ENHANCING INTERVENTIONS

Researchers evaluated a 12-year study of an efficacy enhancing intervention (Lorig & Gonzales, 1992). Patients with arthritis were randomized to one of four groups: (a) exercise; (b) pain management; (c) both exercise and pain management; and (d) a waiting list. Trained intervenors in the three intervention groups used techniques consistent with Bandura's (1997) description of sources of efficacy information to increase participants' perceptions of self-efficacy; participants on the waiting list did not interact with intervenors.

Because intervention programs involving training that included goal-setting and stress-reduction strategies achieved more positive results than purely supportive interventions (Telch & Telch, 1986), goal-setting and stress-reduction strategies were included in the Lorig and Gonzalez (1992) study. Significant improvements in participants' pain, disability, and health status were reported in each of the three intervention groups four months after the intervention suggesting that efficacy-enhancing interventions delivered by trained intervenors may contribute to favorable clinical outcomes. Randomized controls in the original studies crossed over at 4 months to participate in the intervention, consequently there were no controls from the original study for comparison at the 4-year follow-up (O'Leary, Shoor, Lorig, & Holman, 1988) or 12-year follow-up (Lorig & Gonzalez, 1992). In an early study intervenors met with participants on five occasions (Lorig, Mazonson, & Holman, 1993); researchers in a later trial increased the number of occasions to seven occasions and reported that attendance fell off (O'Leary, Shoor, Lorig, & Holman, 1988).

## PURPOSE

The diagnosis and treatment of breast cancer affects patients' quality of life, symptom distress, and self-care self-efficacy. The aims of this study were to conduct a randomized field experiment to test the effects of a self-efficacy intervention delivered on five occasions and designed to enhance patients' self-care self-efficacy. Dependent measures, quality of life, symptom distress, and self-care self-efficacy were assessed at three time points (baseline, 4 months, and 8 months post-chemotherapy). The hypotheses were that at 4 months and 8 months after participants began chemotherapy (a) the efficacy-enhancing experimental group would have significantly higher scores on quality of life and self-care self-efficacy than the control group; and (b) the efficacy-enhancing group would have significantly less symptom distress than the control group. The intervention was expected to influence behaviors by enhancing patients' cognitive appraisals of perceived self-care self-efficacy.

## METHOD

### Sample and Procedures

Participants were recruited from four settings in New Jersey where chemotherapy for cancer was administered. A contact person in each agency notified a recruiter when eligible new patients began treatment. The recruiter visited the agency to explain the study to the patient and ask for informed consent in accordance with approved IRB protocol in each setting.

Patients consenting to participate in the study were 56 women within the first cycle of beginning chemotherapy for Stage I or Stage II breast cancer who were 18 to 70 years of age, able to speak and read English, and not diagnosed with a cancer of the brain or a major psychiatric disorder as defined in the DSM-IV (1994). Women completed study questionnaires in the treatment setting for the initial data collection (baseline) and the four-month follow-up; they completed the eight-month follow-up questionnaires by mail.

Patients were randomized to two groups: the efficacy-enhancing experimental group and the control group. Both groups received the usual preparation, which included being told that medications would be given on specific days, that side effects might occur, and that medications to control the side effects could be given. The control group received a booklet, "Cancer Chemotherapy and Care." The

**Table 8.1.** Application of self-efficacy theory to interventions.

| Sources of self-efficacy (Bandura, 1997) | Relationship of interventions to sources of self-efficacy |
|---|---|
| Performance accomplishments | Participant contracts to practice specific self-care behaviors |
| | RA gives positive feedback for participants' accomplishments |
| Vicarious experience | Participant views videotape |
| Verbal persuasion | RA asserts patient has capability for success |
| | RA gives verbal encouragement for self-care activities |
| Physiological states | RA reinterprets patients' expression of stress |
| | RA provides realistic symptom interpretation |
| | RA maintains a calm attitude |

*Note.* RA: research assistants were intervenors in this study.

booklet, written at a ninth grade reading level, incorporated information about cancer and normal cells regarding cell division, cell generation cycles, and the rationale for combination chemotherapy.

## Intervention

The efficacy intervention group (a) viewed a 5-minute videotape; (b) received the "Self-Care Behaviors" booklet that incorporated elements of the social cognition model; and (c) received five efficacy-enhancing counseling interventions delivered in monthly 1:1 sessions by trained intervenors. Intervenors, nurses attending a graduate program in nursing, were familiar with cancer diagnosis and treatment. An 8-hour training program given by the principal investigator (E. L.) focused on teaching efficacy-enhancing techniques to ensure that theory-based counseling interventions were congruent with the Bandura (1997) framework. Examples of self-efficacy enhancing techniques and strategies used by patients have been described (Lev & Owen, 2000). The relationship of the interventions to the Bandura (1997) framework is shown in Table 8.1. Interventions were audiotaped and the principal investigator reviewed audiotapes to ensure that intervenors were following study protocol.

The videotape, designed by the principal investigator (PI) and consultants (Lev, Paul, & Papianni, 1996), showed three survivors of breast cancer who successfully used self-care behaviors to prevent side effects. Each survivor was asked to describe her diagnosis of breast cancer, what she did to help herself, the worst part of the experience, how she dealt with her worst times, the best part of the experience, what she would like to tell other women going through treatment for breast cancer, and how the experience of breast cancer changed her life. The implication was that survivors were able to exert influence over aspects of their treatment.

Self-care behaviors were described in the "Self-Care Behaviors" booklets, which were written at a ninth grade reading level. The booklet included self-care behaviors such as attention refocusing, imagery, dissociation, reframing, and self-encouragement. Participants were asked to read the booklet and contract to set their own goals regarding practice of specific self-care behaviors.

## Measures

*Quality of Life.* The Functional Assessment of Cancer Treatment-Breast (FACT-B, Version 2), composed of 43 items, was used to measure quality of life (Cella et al., 1993). The FACT-B was chosen for this study, as items were systematically developed, represent a range of important aspects of quality of life as indicated by patient review, and include the 33 items in the FACT as well as 10 items specific to people with breast cancer. Items specific to persons with breast cancer included the following:

1. Assessing possible physical symptoms due to side effects of the medications ("I have been bothered by hair loss"; "I am bothered by a change in weight");
2. Physical symptoms due to side effects of surgical treatment ("My arms are swollen or tender");
3. Psychological factors ("I am self-conscious about the way I dress"; and "I am able to feel like a woman").

The reported internal consistency (coefficient alpha) for the FACT ranged from .65 to .82. The correlation between the total score on the FACT and the Functional Living Index-Cancer (Schipper, Clinch, McMurray, & Levitt, 1984) was .79, indicating that the FACT is related to another instrument that has been used to measure quality of life, well-being, and activity level. The FACT was able to differentiate patients according to stage of disease (I, II, III, IV). The measurement system, under development since 1987, moved into its fourth version in November, 1997 (Cella, 1997).

The quality of life score of the FACT-B, version 2, comprised six subscale scores: physical well-being, social/family well-being, relationship with doctor, emotional well-being, functional well-being, and additional concerns. Participants were asked to respond to each item using a 5-point response scale ranging from "Not At All" to "Very Much." Sample items were, "I have a lack of energy," and "My work (include work in home) is fulfilling." The FACT-B is scored by reversing negatively worded items and summing responses to yield a total score.

*Symptom Distress.* McCorkle and Young (1978) developed the Symptom Distress Scale (SDS) to measure degree of distress associated with patients' symptoms. The alpha reliability for the total scale was 0.82 for 53 patients with chronic illness and validity evidence was reported by McCorkle and Young (1978). The SDS discriminated cancer patients from heart patient survivors and home care patients from controls; it detected changes in patients' symptoms at the completion of treatment and during active tumor growth and detected little or no change in scores of patients whose condition remained stable (McCorkle & Benoliel, 1983; McCorkle, Benoliel, Donaldson, & Goodell, 1986; McCorkle, Robinson, Nuamah, Lev, & Benoliel, 1998). The SDS measures physical symptoms such as nausea, appetite, insomnia, pain, bowel patterns, breathing, cough, and psychological factors such as concentration, appearance, mood, and outlook. Respondents are asked to rate each item using a 5-point response format ranging from 1 (normal or no distress) to 5 (extensive distress). Total symptom distress is obtained as the unweighted sum of the 13 scales, a value that could range from 13 to 65, with higher scores denoting greater levels of symptom distress.

*Self-Care Self-Efficacy.* Self-care self-efficacy, the individual's confidence in using strategies to promote health, was measured by Strategies Used by Patients to Promote Health (SUPPH), a self-report instrument (Lev & Owen, 1996). Internal consistency reliability and validity data were reported for patients diagnosed with cancer, receiving hemodialysis for End Stage Renal Disease, and after a cerebral vascular accident (Lev & Owen, 1996; Lev & Owen, 1998; Lev, Paul, & Owen, 1999; Robinson-Smith, Johnston, & Allen, 2000). Item examples for each of the four factors are:

1. Coping (e.g., "Keeping my stress within healthy limits");
2. Stress Reduction (e.g., "Practicing stress reduction techniques even when I'm feeling sick");
3. Making Decisions (e.g., "Choosing among treatment alternatives recommended by my physician the one that seems right for me");
4. Enjoying Life (e.g., "Helping other people going through cancer treatment"). Respondents were asked to rate their degree of confidence in carrying out specific self-care behaviors.

Each item of the SUPPH is rated on a 5-point scale of confidence from 1 = "very little" to 5 = "quite a lot." The instrument is scored by summing responses. Selected biographic data including age, background, religion, marital status, level of education, job, stage of disease and treatment, were provided by the participants.

## RESULTS

### Sample

Fifty-six women were recruited to the study. Because initial data were incomplete for three women, data are reported for 53. Twenty-eight women were randomly assigned to the control group and 25, to the intervention group. Of these, 24 women completed three occasions of data collection; however, 5 had missing data at the 8-month follow-up, and one woman's score was eliminated as an outlier. Data analysis was performed for 18 women (10 intervention and 8 control) with complete data for the three measurement occasions. Reasons for dropout included death (1), homelessness (1), unwillingness to participate in control group (4), development of other cancers (5), could not be located for the 8-month follow-up (9), did not return 8-month follow-up survey (9). Participants ranged in age from 30 to 72, with a mean age of 50 (median = 51); they were mainly White, Catholic, married, and high school graduates. Additional data are shown in Table 8.2.

Due to the small sample, this study is considered a descriptive rather than an inferential study. As such, ANCOVA, a statistical inference tool for assessing unequal starting points, is inappropriate.

## Method of Data Analysis

Measurements of significance are, in part, a function of sample size. Because even trivial effects demonstrate significance under the $p < .05$ criterion if the data set is large enough, many researchers report effect size, a measure of practical signifi- cance (Cohen, 1988). Eta square is one measure of effect size that corresponds to the familiar R squared from regression analysis and ranges from zero to 100% of variance. Cohen (1988) suggested the following guidelines for effect sizes: small (= .01), medium (= .06), and large (= .14). The ANOVA interaction effect is used to investigate change in both experimental and control groups across the three occasions of measurement. The interaction term thus answers whether two groups change in different ways over time (see Table 8.3). Effect sizes are not based on the entire sample, but only on the women who had complete data across the three measurement occasions. Effect sizes do not depict the nature of the interaction; however, inspection of the various interaction plots to which the effect sizes refer, revealed that the efficacy-enhancing experimental group had more positive changes and changed more dramatically over time than the control group. In short, groups generally changed in ways predicted by the hypotheses.

Another approach to investigation of whether or not the change was clinically significant is to calculate Cohen's (1988) "*d*," which refers to how many standard deviations apart average scores are. Cohen's "*d*" is the kind of effect size often reported in studying group differences. For *d*, < 0.30 is small; 0.50 is moderate; and > 0.80 is large (Cohen, 1988). For example, for the intervention group, the *d* value on "coping" between occasion 1 and occasion 3 is .88 standard deviations, or a large effect size. The same calculation for the control group gives a .17 standard deviation change, a small effect size. Thus the "coping" change for the intervention group was substantially larger than the change for the control group.

The measure of effect size, unlike a significance test, also allows comparisons across studies having varied sample size. Powerful findings are produced when

**TABLE 8.2. Description of Study Participants**

|  | *n* | % |
|---|---|---|
| Marital status |  |  |
| Married | 42 | 79 |
| Widowed | 6 | 11 |
| Never married | 2 | 4 |
| Divorced | 2 | 4 |
| Separated | 1 | 2 |
| Background |  |  |
| White | 44 | 83 |
| Black | 8 | 15 |
| Hispanic | 1 | 2 |
| Religion |  |  |
| Catholic | 30 | 57 |
| Protestant | 17 | 32 |
| Jewish | 4 | 7 |
| Other | 2 | 4 |
| Education |  |  |
| No high school | 1 | 2 |
| Some high school | 4 | 7 |
| High school graduate | 20 | 38 |
| Some college | 13 | 25 |
| College graduate | 10 | 19 |
| Graduate school | 5 | 10 |
| Job |  |  |
| Skilled | 31 | 59 |
| Housewife | 9 | 17 |
| Professional | 9 | 17 |
| Retired | 2 | 4 |
| Unskilled | 1 | 2 |
| Disability | 1 | 2 |
| Stage of disease |  |  |
| Stage I | 19 | 36 |
| Stage II | 25 | 47 |
| Not reported | 3 | 6 |
| Surgery |  |  |
| Lumpectomy | 24 | 45 |
| Mastectomy | 20 | 38 |

Note. Missing data are responsible for numbers < sample size.

**TABLE 8.3. Means, Standard Deviations and Eta-Squared for Measures of Control (C) and Intervention (I) Groups Over 3 Occasions**

| | Baseline | | | | Occasion 4-Months | | | | 8-Months | | | | |
| | mean | | SD | | mean | | SD | | mean | | SD | | Eta-Squared |
| Measure | C | I | C | I | C | I | C | I | C | I | C | I | |
|---|---|---|---|---|---|---|---|---|---|---|---|---|---|
| SUPPH | | | | | | | | | | | | | |
| Coping | 4.05 | 3.61 | .56 | .94 | 4.04 | 4.21 | .89 | .47 | 4.13 | 4.17 | .45 | .33 | .089** |
| Stress Reduction | 2.95 | 3.14 | .89 | .87 | 3.40 | 3.86 | 1.07 | .63 | 3.43 | 3.87 | .90 | .73 | .016* |
| Making Decisions | 3.04 | 3.76 | .86 | 1.29 | 3.75 | 4.30 | 1.26 | .63 | 3.58 | 4.13 | .99 | .83 | .005 |
| Enjoying Life | 3.87 | 3.33 | .87 | 1.22 | 4.08 | 4.26 | 1.00 | .86 | 4.25 | 4.23 | .54 | .42 | .064** |
| SDS | 1.49 | 1.83 | .26 | .70 | 1.39 | 1.30 | .26 | .28 | 1.31 | 1.27 | .24 | .24 | .140*** |
| FACT | | | | | | | | | | | | | |
| Physical | 3.41 | 2.91 | .26 | .23 | 3.59 | 3.50 | .19 | .17 | 3.73 | 3.70 | .13 | .12 | .072** |
| Social | 3.64 | 3.44 | .14 | .13 | 3.49 | 3.37 | .15 | .13 | 3.36 | 3.57 | .22 | .19 | .110** |
| MD relationship | 3.69 | 3.50 | .22 | .19 | 3.56 | 3.65 | .19 | .17 | 3.81 | 3.50 | .18 | .16 | .075*** |
| Emotional | 3.33 | 3.20 | .24 | .22 | 3.35 | 3.52 | .19 | .17 | 3.60 | 3.56 | .16 | .15 | .048* |
| Functional | 3.00 | 2.98 | .25 | .22 | 3.20 | 3.43 | .17 | .15 | 3.35 | 3.47 | .23 | .20 | .031* |
| Additional Concerns | 2.79 | 2.45 | .26 | .23 | 2.78 | 2.78 | .21 | .19 | 2.92 | 2.69 | .22 | .20 | .063** |

*small effect size (.01); **medium effect size (.06); ***large effect size (.14).

small positive effect sizes are consistent across many studies and generalizability is possible through meta-analytic aggregation (Devine & Westlake, 1995; Kinney, Burfitt, Stullenbarger, Rees, & Debolt, 1996; Lipsey, 1990; Meyer & Mark, 1995; Tobler, 1994; Whatley & Milne, 1998).

## Descriptive Statistics

At 4 and 8 months the interaction effects for the FACT-B ranged from small for functional well-being (eta square = .03) to large for social/family well-being (eta square = .110); effects for the SDS were large (eta square = .140); and for factors on the SUPPH, effect sizes ranged from small (eta square = .01) for Enjoying Life and Stress Reduction to medium (eta square = .089) for Coping, and large (eta square = .141) for Making Decisions. The greatest changes in outcome measures occurred between baseline and 4 months, and changes were sustained in the 8-month follow-up period. Additional data are shown in Table 2.

## DISCUSSION

Results supported the hypotheses: At 4 months and 8 months after women began chemotherapy scores for the women in the efficacy-enhancing group had increased on measures of quality of life and self-care self-efficacy had decreased on the measure of symptom distress. Due to the small number of women who had completed data across three measurement occasions, this report is considered a pilot study, that is, it is meant to be heuristic, to suggest directions for future data collections and intervention.

Nurses provided interventions congruent with the theoretical basis of self-efficacy. The study provided support for the hypotheses that efficacy-enhancing interventions enhance patients' quality of life and decrease patients' symptoms. Efficacy enhancing interventions may provide cancer patients with the means to participate in self-care activities, supporting Orem's (1995) assertions that nursing care includes providing patients with self-care strategies. Results support Merluzzi and Sanchez (1997a, 1997b) who asserted that health care providers' understanding of patients' self-efficacy expectations may facilitate patients' coping with cancer.

These data are consistent with data suggesting that psychosocial intervention reduces psychologic distress and symptoms and increases quality of life in patients with breast cancer (Andersen, 1992; Baider, Uziely, & NeNour, 1994; Fawzy & Fawzy, 1994; Greer et al., 1992; Longman, Braden, & Mishel, 1996; Meyer & Mark, 1995; Trijsburg, van Knippenberg, & Pijpma, 1992; Whatley & Milne, 1998). Also supported are Musci and Dodd's (1990) finding that self-care behaviors can be learned and Longman and associates' (1996) suggestion that women who practice self-care strategies experience fewer side effects. Bandura (1997) described self-efficacy as the exercise of control, and control has been identified as a mediator of successful adjustment in cancer patients (Cunningham, Lockwood, & Cunningham, 1991).

Nurses who were research assistants in this study provided interventions to patients. Researchers suggest that psychosocial interventions may affect how one deals with stress as well as one's survival (Fawzy, Fawzy, Arndt, & Pasnau, 1995; Greer, 1995; Greer et al., 1992; Spiegel, 1997). Yet previous researchers reported that nurses were more likely than physicians to support psychosocial interventions for breast cancer patients (Del Giudice, Leszcz, Pritchard, Vincent, & Goodwin, 1997; Walker & Eremin, 1996). In centers offering counseling for cancer patients, psychosocial support services were provided by clinical social workers 84% of the time, by nurses 79% of the time, and by psychologists 71% of the time (Coluzzi et al., 1995).

The study described in this chapter included patients diagnosed with either Stage I or Stage II breast cancer. Walker and associates (1999) studied 96 women with advanced breast cancer. The hypotheses that patients randomized to relaxation and guided imagery would have greater quality of life and improved coping skills, were supported. Immunological differences between experimental and control groups were noted, demonstrating biological as well as psychosocial effects of the intervention (Walker et al., 1999).

## Limitations of the Study

The small sample size was a major limitation of the study. Recruitment proceeded more slowly than anticipated although additional sites were added. In one site the contact person did not notify recruiters about eligible new patients despite periodic reminders. A merger between hospitals may have contributed to limited participation in two sites. Referrals to the study may have been negatively affected by changes in the health care system in participating settings. Attrition was primarily affected by the fact that participants who moved their residence after completing chemotherapy treatment were frequently unable to be located and, therefore, were lost to the study.

Nurse researchers employed primarily by educational institutions not affiliated with health care agencies have experienced political and procedural obstacles in gaining access to potential research participants within health care agencies (Nokes & Dolan, 1992). Adding a coinvestigator who is employed by the health care agency may facilitate access to participants (Nokes & Dolan, 1992).

Previous researchers reported that participant accrual for cancer patients resulted in from 30% to 69% of eligible patients participating in the study (Burton et al., 1995; Motzer, Moseley, & Lewis, 1997; Richardson, Post-White, Singletary, & Justice, 1998). Attrition rates for longitudinal studies ranged from 17% to 25% (Abraham, Chalifoux & Evers, 1991; Motzer, Moseley, & Lewis, 1997; Yanagihara, Harvey, McLarty, & Genoway, 1990). Motzer and associates (1997) suggested specific strategies to increase sample size of a randomized trial of a nursing intervention with breast cancer patients. Several student research assistants worked on the study reported in this article for varying amounts of time and several hospitals were depended upon to facilitate recruitment. The fact that many people were involved in the study may have resulted in clinical relationships compromised by inconsistent patterns of communication.

## Implications for Intervention

In a study by Coluzzi and associates (1995) 10% of National Cancer Institute-designated cancer centers did not offer counseling services and funding for psychosocial interventions has decreased (Anderson, 1992) despite overwhelming evidence of improved quality of life and adjustment in cancer patients who do receive counseling. In this study the greatest changes in quality of life, self-care, self-efficacy and symptom distress occurred between baseline and 4 months after beginning chemotherapy. Without intervention cancer patients' measures of quality of life and self-care self-efficacy decreased and symptom distress increased (Lev, Paul, & Owen, 1999). Therefore psychosocial intervention should begin as early as feasible. There is little direct evidence of cost/benefit data associated with counseling cancer patients; however, possible savings may include reduced physician visits as well as reduced use of pharmacologic interventions for patients who receive counseling (Whatley & Milne, 1998).

Patients' self-efficacy could be assessed using instruments measuring self-efficacy in cancer patients. Assessment of self-efficacy could be an aspect of the care given by health professionals (Lev, 1995). Interventions could be designed to be given in areas in which individual patients demonstrate need. For example, if a patient's coping ability were low, interventions could be given to enhance coping.

## Conclusions and Future Research

Psychosocial support needs to be available for women with breast cancer in order to increase their quality of life and decrease symptoms. Evidence that biologic changes may accompany psychosocial changes suggests that further study of psychosocial interventions for cancer patients should include biological measures. Future studies of breast cancer patients should include patients with more advanced cancers as well as patients in early stages.

No attempt was made to separate components of the intervention given in this study. Psychosocial interventions and videotapes have each contributed to positive health outcomes for patients (Fawzy, Fawzy, Arndt, & Pasnau, 1995; Gagliano, 1988; Robinson et al., 1997; Whatley & Milne, 1998). It would be beneficial to understand whether benefits could be achieved with the videotape alone or whether it is necessary to deliver the intervention individually in order for patients to achieve positive outcomes. It would also be beneficial to know whether or not a telephone intervention rather than a face-to-face meeting would be sufficient for patients to achieve positive outcomes.

# REFERENCES

Abraham, I. L., Chalifoux, Z. L., & Evers, G. C. M. (1991, September). *Conditions, interventions, and outcomes: A quantitative analysis of nursing research.* Paper presented at the Patient Outcomes Research Conference sponsored by the National Center for Nursing Research, National Institutes of Health, Rockville, MD.

American Psychiatric Association. (1994). *DSM IV: Diagnostic and Statistical Manual of Mental Disorders* (4th ed.). Washington, DC: Author.

Andersen, B. L. (1992). Psychological interventions for cancer patients to enhance the quality of life. *Journal of Consulting and Clinical Psychology, 60*(4), 552-568.

Andrykowski, M. A., Greiner, C. B., Altmaier, E. M., Burish, T. G., Antin, J. H., Gingrich, R., McGarigle, C., & Henslee-Downey, P. J. (1995). Quality of life following bone marrow transplantation: Findings from a multicentre study. *British Journal of Cancer, 71*(6), 1322-1399.

Baider, L., Uziely, B., & DeNour, A. K. (1994). Progressive muscle relaxation and guided imagery in cancer patients. *General Hospital Psychiatry, 16,* 340-347.

Bandura, A. (1997). *Self-efficacy: The exercise of control.* New York: Freeman.

Beck, K. H., & Lund, A. K. (1981). The effects of health threat seriousness and personal efficacy upon intentions and behavior. *Journal of Applied Social Psychology, 11,* 401-415.

Burish, R. G., & Redd, W. H. (1994). Symptom control in psychosocial oncology. *Cancer, 74*(4 Suppl. 4), 1438-1444.

Burish, T. G., Snyder, S. L., & Jenkins, R. A. (1991). Preparing patients for cancer chemotherapy: Effect of coping preparation and relaxation interventions. *Journal of Consulting and Clinical Psychology, 39*(4), 518-515.

Burton, M. V., Parker, R. W., Farrell, A., Bailey, D., Conneely, J., Booth, S., & Elcombe, S. (1995). A randomized controlled trial of preoperative psychological preparation for mastectomy. *Psycho-Oncology, 4,* 1-19.

Carey, M. P., & Burish, T. G. (1988). Etiology and treatment of the psychological side effects associated with cancer chemotherapy: A critical review and discussion. *Psychological Bulletin, 104*(3), 307-325.

Cella, D. (1997). *FACIT Manual: Manual of the Functional Assessment of Chronic Illness Therapy (FACIT) Measurement System.* Evanston, IL: Evanston Northwestern Healthcare and Northwestern University, Center on Outcomes, Research and Education.

Cella, D. F., Tulsky, G. S., Gray, G., Sarafian, B., Linn, E., Bonomi, A., Silberman, M., Yellen, S.B., Winicour, P., Brannon, J., Eckberg, K., Lloyd, S., Purl, S., Blendowski, C., Goodman, M., Barnicle, M., Stewart, I., McHale, M., Bonomi, P., Kaplan, E., Taylor, S., Thomas, C. R., & Harris, J. (1993). The functional assessment of cancer therapy scale: Development and validation of the general measure. *Journal of Clinical Oncology, 11,* 570-579.

Cohen, J. (1988). *Statistical power analysis for the behavioral sciences* (2nd ed.). Hillsdale, NJ: Lawrence Erlbaum Associates.

Coluzzi, P. H., Grant, M., Doroshow, J. H., Rhiner, M., Ferrell, B., & Rivera, L. (1995). Survey of the provision of supportive care services at National Cancer Institute-designated cancer centers. *Journal of Clinical Oncology, 13*(3), 756-764.

Creagan, E. T. (1993). Psychosocial issues in oncologic practice. *Mayo Clinic Proceedings, 68*(2), 161-167.

Cunningham, A. J., Edmonds, C. V. I., & Williams, D. (1999). Delivering a very brief psychoeducational program to cancer patients and family members in a large group format. *Psycho-Oncology, 8,* 177-182.

Cunningham, A. J., Lockwood, G. A., & Cunningham, J. A. (1991). A relationship between perceived self-efficacy and quality of life in cancer patients. *Patient Education and Counseling, 17,* 71-78.

Del Giudice, M. E., Leszcz, M., Pritchard, K. I., Vincent, L., & Goodwin, P. (1997). Attitudes of Canadian oncology practitioners toward psychosocial interventions in clinical and research settings in women with breast cancer. *Psycho-Oncology, 6,* 178-189.

Demark-Wahnefried, W., Winer, E. P., & Rimer, B. K. (1993). Why women gain weight with adjuvant chemotherapy for breast cancer. *Journal of Clinical Oncology, 11*(7), 1418-1429.

Devine, E. C., & Westlake, S. K. (1995). The effects of psychoeducational care provided to adults with cancer: Meta-analysis of 116 studies. *Oncology Nursing Forum, 22*(9), 1369-1381.

Dodd, M. (1984). Self-care for patients with breast cancer to prevent side effects of chemotherapy: A concern for public health nursing. *Public Health Nursing, 1*(4), 202-209.

Edgar, L., Rosberger, Z., & Nowlis, D. (1992). Coping with cancer during the first year after diagnosis. *Cancer, 69*(3), 817-828.

Edmonds, C. V., Lockwood, G. A., & Cunningham, A. J. (1999). Psychological response to long-term group therapy: A randomized trial with metastatic breast cancer patients. *Psycho-Oncology, 8*(1), 74-91.

Fawzy, F. I. (1995). A short-term psychoeducational intervention for patients newly diagnosed with cancer. *Supportive Care in Cancer, 3*(4), 235-238.

Fawzy, R. I., & Fawzy, N. W. (1994). A structured psychoeducational intervention for cancer patients. *General Hospital Psychiatry, 16*(3), 149-192.

Fawzy, F. I., Fawzy, N. W., Arndt, L. A., & Pasnau, R. O. (1995). Critical review of psychosocial interventions in cancer care. *Archives of General Psychiatry, 52*(2), 100-113.

Ferrans, C. E. (1990). Development of a quality of life index for patients with cancer. *Oncology Nursing Forum, 17*(3), 15-19.

Ferrell, B. R., Grant, M., Funk, B., Garcia, N., Otis-Green, S., & Schaffner, M. L. (1996). Quality of life in breast cancer. *Cancer Practice, 4*(6), 331-340.

Ferrell, B., Wisdom, C., Wenzl, C., & Brown, J. (1989). Effects of controlled-release morphine on quality of life for cancer pain. *Oncology Nursing Forum, 16*(4), 521-526.

Gagliano, M. E. (1988). A literature review on the efficacy of video in patient education. *Journal of Medical Education, 63,* 785-792.

Greer, S. (1995). Improving quality of life: Adjuvant psychological therapy for patients with cancer. *Supportive Care in Cancer, 3*(4), 248-251.

Greer, S., Morrey, S., Baruch, J. D. R., Watson, M., Robertson, B. M., Mason, A., Rowden, L., Law, M. G., & Bliss, J. M. (1992). Adjuvant psychologic therapy for patients with cancer: A prospective randomized trial. *British Medical Journal, 304,* 676-680.

Kinney, M. R., Burfitt, S. N., Stullenbarger, E., Rees, B., & Debolt, M. R. (1996). Quality of life in cardiac patient research: A meta-analysis. *Nursing Research, 45*(3), 173-180.

Lev, E. L. (1992). Patients' strategies for adapting to cancer treatment. *Western Journal of Nursing Research, 14*(5), 595-617.

Lev, E. L. (1995). Theoretical linkages and outcomes in a nursing intervention study using triangulation. *Clinical Nurse Specialist, 9*(6), 300-305.

Lev, E. L. (1997). Bandura's theory of self-efficacy: Applications to oncology. *Scholarly Inquiry for Nursing Practice,11*(1), 21-37.

Lev, E. L., & Owen, S. V. (1996) A measure of self-care self-efficacy. *Research in Nursing & Health, 19,* 421-429.

Lev, E. L., & Owen, S. V. (1998). A prospective study of adjustment to hemodialysis. *American Nephrology Nurses Association (ANNA) Journal, 25*(5), 495-506.

Lev, E. L., & Owen, S. V. (2000). Counseling women with breast cancer using principles developed by Albert Bandura. *Perspectives in Psychiatric Care, 36*(4), 131-138.

Lev, E. L., Paul, D., & Owen, S. V. (1999). Age, self-efficacy, and change in patients' adjustments to cancer. *Cancer Practice, 7*(4), 170-176.

Lev, E. L., Paul, D. B., & Papianni, M. (Producers). (1996). *The breast cancer journey: Mission possible* (video). (Available from E. Lev, Rutgers College of Nursing, 180 University Ave., Newark, NJ 07102).

Lipsey, M. W. (1990). *Design sensitivity: Statistical power for experimental research.* Newbury Park, CA: Sage.

Longman, A. J., Braden, C. J., & Mishel, M. H. (1996). Side effects burden in women with breast cancer. *Cancer Practice, 4*(5), 274-280.

Lorig, K., & Gonzalez, V. (1992). The integration of theory with practice: A 12-year case study. *Health Education Quarterly, 19*(3), 355-368.

Lorig, K. R., Mazonson, P. D., & Holman, H. R. (1993). Evidence suggesting that health education for self-management in patients with chronic arthritis has sustained health benefits while reducing health care costs. *Arthritis and Rheumatism, 36*(4), 439-446.

McCorkle, R., & Benoliel, J. Q. (1983). Symptom distress, current concerns, and mood disturbance after diagnosis of life-threatening disease. *Social Science & Medicine, 17,* 431-438.

McCorkle, R., Benoliel, J. Q., Donaldson, G., & Goodell, B. (1986). *Evaluation of cancer management* (Grant # NU 01001). Final report of project supported by the Division of Nursing, Bureau of Health Professions, Health Resources and Services Administration, U.S. Public Health Service. Seattle, WA: Community Health Care Systems Department, University of Washington.

McCorkle, R., Robinson, L., Nuamah, I., Lev, E., & Benoliel, J. Q. (1998). The effects of home nursing care for patients during terminal illness on the bereaved's psychological distress. *Nursing Research, 47*(1), 2-10.

McCorkle, R., & Young, K. (1978). Development of a symptom distress scale. *Cancer Nursing, 1,* 373-378.

Merluzzi, T. V., & Sanchez, M. A. M. (1997a). Assessment of self-efficacy and coping with cancer: Development and validation of the cancer behavior inventory. *Health Psychology, 16*(2), 163-170.

Merluzzi, T.V., & Sanchez, M. A. M. (1997b). Perceptions of coping behaviors by persons with cancer and health care providers. *Psycho-Oncology, 6,* 197-203.

Meyer, T. J., & Mark, M. M. (1995). Effects of psychosocial interventions with adult cancer patients: A meta-analysis of randomised experiments. *Health Psychology, 14*(2), 101-108.

Motzer, S. A., Moseley, J. R., & Lewis, F. M. (1997). Recruitment and retention of families in clinical trials with longitudinal designs. *Western Journal of Nursing Research, 19*(3), 314-333.

Musci, E. C., & Dodd, M. J. (1990). Predicting self-care with patients and family members' affective states and family functioning. *Oncology Nursing Forum, 17*(3), 394-400.

Nokes, K. M., & Dolan, M. S. (1992). Experiences of nurse-researchers in gaining access to subjects for clinical nursing research. *Journal of Professional Nursing, 8*(2), 115-119.

O'Leary, A., Shoor, S., Lorig, K., & Holman, H. (1988). A cognitive-behavioral treatment for rheumatoid arthritis. *Health Psychology, 7*(6), 527-544.

Orem, D. (1995). *Nursing: Concepts of practice* (5th ed.). St. Louis, MO: Mosby-Year Book, Inc.

Richardson, M. A., Post-White, J., Singletary, S. E., & Justice, B. (1998). Recruitment for complementary/alternative medicine trials: Who participates after breast cancer. *Annuals of Behavioral Medicine, 20*(3), 190-198.

Robinson, P., Katon, W., Von Korff, M., Bush, T., Simon, G., Lin, E., & Walker, E. (1997). The education of depressed primary care patients: What do patients think of interactive booklets and a video. *The Journal of Family Practice, 44*(6), 562-571.

Robinson-Smith, G., Johnston, M. V., & Allen, J. (in press). Self-care self-efficacy, quality of life and depression after stroke. *Archives of Physical Medicine and Rehabilitation, 18,* 460-464.

Schipper, H., Clinch, J., McMurray, A., & Levitt, M. (1984). Measuring the quality of life of cancer patients: The Functional Living Index-Cancer: Development and validation. *Journal of Clinical Oncology, 2,* 472-483.

Spiegel, D. (1997). Psychosocial aspects of breast cancer treatment. *Seminars in Oncology, 24*(Suppl. 1), 36-47.

Telch, C. F., & Telch, M. J. (1986). Group coping skills instruction and supportive group therapy for cancer patients: A comparison of strategies. *Journal of Consulting and Clinical Psychology, 54*(6), 802-808.

Tobler, N. (1994). Meta-analytical issues for prevention intervention research. *National Institute of Drug Abuse Research Monograph, 142,* 342-403.

Trijsburg, R. W., van Knipenberg, F. C. E., & Pijpma, S. E. (1992). Effects of psychologic treatment on cancer patients: A critical review. *Psychosomatic Medicine, 54,* 489-517.

Vasterling, J., Jenkins, R. A., Tope, D. M., & Burish, T. G. (1993). Cognitive distraction and relaxation training for the control of side effects due to cancer chemotherapy. *Journal of Behavioral Medicine. 16*(1), 65-80.

Walker, L. G., & Eremin, O. (1996). Psychological assessment and intervention: Future prospects for women with breast cancer. *Seminars in Surgical Oncology, 12*(1), 76-83.

Walker, L. G., Walker, M. B., Ogston, K., Heys, S. D., Ah-See, A. K., Miller, I. D., Hutcheon, A. W., Sarkar, T. K., & Eremin, O. (1999). Psychological, clinical and pathological effects of relaxation training and guided imagery during primary chemotherapy. *British Journal of Cancer, 80*(1-2), 262-268.

Whatley, P., & Milne, R. (1998). *Psychosocial interventions in oncology counselling services for women with breast cancer* (Development & Evaluation Committee Report No. 86). Bristol, UK: South and West Regional Health Authority. Available: www.epi.bris.ac.uk/rd/publicat/dec

Yanagihara, R., Harvey, C., McLarty, J., & Genoway, P. (1990) Subject accrual, retention, and attrition on a lung cancer chemoprevention trial. *Proceedings of the Annual Meeting of the American Society of Clinical Oncology, 9,* A237.

*Acknowledgments.* Research for this chapter was funded by R15 CA 63590-01A2, awarded to Elise L. Lev and from the Institutional Minority Student Development Program: Grant Number 1 R25 GM 0826-02.

# Index